Cassandra L. Verdi, MPH, RD, and Stephanie A. Dunbar, MPH, RD

DIABETES SUPERFOODS——
——Cookbook and Meal Planner

Power-Packed Recipes and Meal Plans Designed to Help You Lose Weight and
Manage Your Blood Glucose

**MORE THAN 110
DIABETES-FRIENDLY RECIPES**

**40 DAYS OF MEAL PLANS
& PRACTICAL TIME-SAVING TIPS**

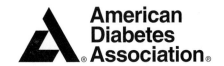

American
Diabetes
Association®

Associate Publisher, Books, Abe Ogden; *Director, Book Operations,* Victor Van Beuren; *Associate Director, Books,* John Clark; *Associate Director, Book Marketing,* Annette Reape; *Senior Manager, Book Editing,* Lauren Wilson; *Project Manager,* Amnet Systems; *Composition,* Amnet Systems; *Cover Design,* Jenn French Designs*; Food Photographer,* Mittera Creative; *Printer,* Marquis Printing.

Printed in Canada
1 3 5 7 9 10 8 6 4 2

The suggestions and information contained in this publication are generally consistent with the *Standards of Medical Care in Diabetes* and other policies of the American Diabetes Association, but they do not represent the policy or position of the Association or any of its boards or committees. Reasonable steps have been taken to ensure the accuracy of the information presented. However, the American Diabetes Association cannot ensure the safety or efficacy of any product or service described in this publication. Individuals are advised to consult a physician or other appropriate health care professional before undertaking any diet or exercise program or taking any medication referred to in this publication. Professionals must use and apply their own professional judgment, experience, and training and should not rely solely on the information contained in this publication before prescribing any diet, exercise, or medication. The American Diabetes Association—its officers, directors, employees, volunteers, and members—assumes no responsibility or liability for personal or other injury, loss, or damage that may result from the suggestions or information in this publication.

Madelyn Wheeler conducted the internal review of this book to ensure that it meets American Diabetes Association guidelines.

♾ The paper in this publication meets the requirements of the ANSI Standard Z39.48-1992 (permanence of paper).

ADA titles may be purchased for business or promotional use or for special sales. To purchase more than 50 copies of this book at a discount, or for custom editions of this book with your logo, contact the American Diabetes Association at the address below or at booksales@diabetes.org.

American Diabetes Association
2451 Crystal Drive, Suite 900
Arlington, VA 22202

Library of Congress Cataloging-in-Publication Data

Names: Verdi, Cassandra L., author. | Dunbar, Stephanie A., author.
Title: Diabetes superfoods cookbook and meal planner : power-packed recipes
    and meal plans designed to help you lose weight and manage your blood
    glucose / Cassandra Verdi, MPH, RD and Stephanie Dunbar, MPH, RD.
Description: Arlington : American Diabetes Association, [2019] | Includes
    index.
Identifiers: LCCN 2018022502 | ISBN 9781580406796 (alk. paper)
Subjects: LCSH: Diabetes—Diet therapy—Recipes. | LCGFT: Cookbooks.
Classification: LCC RC662 .V46 2019 | DDC 641.5/6314—dc23
LC record available at https://lccn.loc.gov/2018022502

Dedication

To my husband, Jimmy, and my daughters, Abigail, Emma, and Scarlett, who have been on this cookbook-writing journey with me since it started over a year ago. Thank you for keeping me smiling, motivated, and inspired to cook healthfully for our family—even on the busiest of days.

—Cassie

To Rose, who challenged my taste buds decades ago, introduced me to superfoods long before they were cool, and motivated me with many creative cooking ideas. And most importantly, thank you for your friendship, your encouragement, and for inspiring many culinary journeys.

—Stephanie

Contents

Acknowledgments

We'd like to recognize our longtime friends at the American Diabetes Association, Victor Van Beuren and Abe Ogden, for their friendship and mentorship throughout the process of writing this book. We are so grateful to have had the opportunity to write a second book in partnership with the Association.

Thank you also to Bekah Renshaw, who was instrumental to the development of this book, and to our meticulous copyeditor, Lauren Wilson, as well as our designer, Amnet Systems, and food photographer, Mittera Creative. And of course, thanks to Lyn Wheeler for her always-detailed recipe analysis and counsel throughout the recipe and meal plan development process. We could not have asked for a better team in compiling this collection of nutritious, flavor-packed recipes and meal plans.

To my parents, Tim and Eileen Rico, my sisters, Katie and Caroline, and my brother-in-law Brent—thank you for all of your unwavering support. I could not have completed this book during my first year of motherhood without your expert taste buds and babysitting help. Thank you also to all of my Chicago friends who shared meals with our family over the last year and served as taste-testers—some of whom may not have known it!

—Cassie

To my son Matthew—thank you for your understanding when the kitchen was in action and there was little space or time for anything but a simple sandwich. You brighten my every day and add joy to life. Thank you also to my family and friends, near and far, who cheer me on with unwavering support not only during the writing of this book, but in life in general.

—Stephanie

Diabetes Superfood:
A food rich in nutrients that benefit diabetes management or nutrients that are typically lacking in the American diet.

What This Book Is All About: A Note from the Authors

Today, it is rare to not know someone whose life has been affected by diabetes. Whether it's your family member, friend, colleague, or even yourself—this chronic disease touches most of us in some way. It's serious. It's life-changing. A diabetes diagnosis means paying close attention to what you eat, what's in your food, and how it's made.

But it does NOT mean you can't enjoy flavorful, delicious meals alongside your family and friends. Food is not only an integral part of our day, but a part of who we are. It sparks memories, it fosters togetherness, and it connects us to our loved ones.

As two registered dietitians with nearly 30 years of collective experience in nutrition and diabetes, this is the reason we're bringing this book to you. Our goal is to show people how deliciously simple eating for diabetes can be when you take a superfoods approach, and to offer easy to make recipes that appeal not only to you, but to the others you dine with.

Keeping this in mind, we've designed many of our recipes to be shared and enjoyed with family and friends. Within these pages, you'll find a practical, holistic approach to eating well, complete with an introduction to nutrition and diabetes (page xiii), our Master Superfoods List (page xvii), and over 110 superfood-infused recipes that meet the American Diabetes Association's recipe guidelines. Then we show you how to put it all together with 40 days of diabetes-friendly meal plans (page 145) so you can see how our recipes (plus additional superfoods) fit into a day of eating.

Our hope is that this book will provide you with the guidance and inspiration you need to better control your diabetes while keeping the joy in mealtime—the superfoods way!

—Cassie and Stephanie

Diabetes and Nutrition 101

How Is Diabetes Managed?

There are many aspects of managing diabetes. Eating well, physical activity, and taking medications, if needed, are key factors. Stress management and adequate sleep are also critical. Of all these factors, for many people, making healthy food choices is the most challenging. What you eat and how much you eat has a direct effect on your blood glucose level, your risk of developing diabetes complications, and many other health factors.

Food is made up of a mix of carbohydrate, protein, and fat. You can think of these as building blocks for your body. Healthy foods not only provide those building blocks, they provide the extra bonus of vitamins, minerals, and fiber. Choosing healthy foods is the best way to give your body the energy it needs to do daily activities and the things that you love!

Following a healthy, balanced meal plan that meets your personal nutrition needs can help you:

- Lower your A1C (average blood glucose over the past 2–3 months)
- Lower your blood pressure
- Improve your cholesterol levels
- Lose weight or maintain your current weight
- Increase your energy level
- Prevent or delay diabetes complications

WHAT ARE THE GENERAL GUIDELINES FOR EATING WELL WITH DIABETES?

- Balance food choices throughout the day across several meals (and snacks, if your meal plan includes them)
- Eat more nonstarchy vegetables
- Choose lean sources of protein
- Choose oils for cooking instead of solid fats
- When eating carbohydrates, choose high-quality carbs like whole grains, dairy foods, beans, and fruit with little to no processing
- Avoid sugary drinks like regular soda, sweet tea, fruit punch, and lemonade
- Cut back on high-calorie snack foods and desserts like chips and cookies

How Do I Plan a Healthy, Balanced Meal?

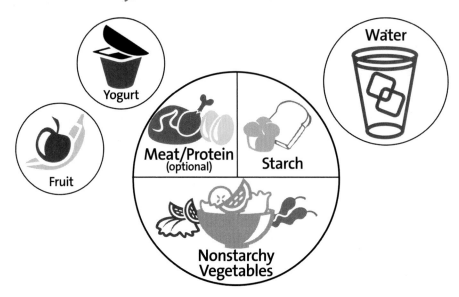

There are several different eating patterns and meal planning tools that are appropriate for people with diabetes. If you've just been diagnosed, the first step is to speak to a healthcare provider to determine your nutritional needs and how much and how often you should be eating. Once you understand what your body needs, you will be ready to plan your meals.

One of the ways to plan a meal is to use the Diabetes Plate Method (pictured above). You don't need any special tools for this portion control method and you don't need to count carbs or calories. It's simple, effective, and you can use it anywhere.

Get started building a healthier plate by following these seven simple steps:

1. Draw an imaginary line across the middle of a 9-inch plate. Then on one half of the plate, draw another line down the middle to give you three sections.
2. Fill the largest section (1/2 of the plate) with nonstarchy vegetables, such as salad, green beans, broccoli, cauliflower, carrots, and tomatoes.
3. In one of the small sections (1/4 of the plate), put starchy foods, such as bread, rice, pasta, corn, beans, and potatoes.
4. The other small section (1/4 of the plate) is for protein foods, such as chicken, fish, lean meat, tofu, and eggs.

5. Add a piece of fruit, a cup of milk or yogurt, or both, as your meal plan allows.

6. Choose healthy fats in small amounts. For cooking, use oils. For salads, some healthy additions are nuts, seeds, avocado, and vinaigrettes.

7. To complete your meal, add a glass of water, unsweetened tea, or coffee.

One of the great things about the Diabetes Plate Method is you can still enjoy your favorite foods by changing how much you eat. Your plate may include more nonstarchy vegetables and less starchy foods, but you're still able to enjoy your favorite foods in the proper portions. The Diabetes Plate Method ensures you have a balance of protein, carbohydrate, and healthy fats at every meal. It also spreads carbohydrate intake throughout the day, which may help manage blood glucose levels.

All of the meal plans in this book are compatible with the Diabetes Plate Method and provide you with examples of balanced meals. Using this method and thinking about the main ingredients in recipes to determine where they fall on the plate can help you create your own meal plans for some of your favorite recipes.

HOW DO I KEEP TRACK OF PORTION SIZES?

Controlling portions can be difficult. The portion sizes of foods and beverages available in packages and served in restaurants have increased significantly over time, making it tough to judge how much to eat. Using the Diabetes Plate Method to control portions is a great place to start. Reading food labels and using measuring cups can be another way to gauge portion sizes.

Using smaller plates, bowls, and glasses can also help keep portions smaller. Measure the plates and glasses in your home. The Diabetes Plate Method suggests using a 9-inch plate; however, many plates now are 12 inches across. The size of drinking glasses also often varies; they can hold up to 12, 16, or even 24 ounces. How much do your glasses hold? Knowing the size of your plates and glasses can help you with portion control.

Use Simple Ways to Estimate Portions
When food labels, measuring cups, or small dishes are not available, use these guidelines to estimate portion sizes:

- 3 ounces of fish, chicken, or meat = 1 deck of cards or a woman's palm
- 1/2 cup = half a baseball
- 1 cup = closed fist or baseball
- 1 tablespoon = thumb
- 1 teaspoon = thumb tip

Our Secret Ingredient? Superfoods!

Pick up any health magazine today, and the odds are high you'll come across a list of top "superfoods." This is a common term in today's world...but what does it actually mean? And can superfoods be a helpful tool for people with diabetes?

The answer is yes, and you're in luck because we've compiled our Master List of Diabetes Superfoods below. Every recipe in this book was developed based on this list and includes one (likely more!) superfood as an ingredient.

Our definition of a diabetes superfood is simple. It's any food that (1) has a nutrient profile beneficial for diabetes management or (2) is rich in key nutrients that are typically lacking in the American diet.

Master List of Diabetes Superfoods

Berries

Strawberries, blackberries, raspberries, blueberries, and cranberries...these little gems are packed with antioxidants, which are cancer-fighting molecules that can remove harmful agents from the body. Berries are also a great source of fiber. We like them fresh, but they can be enjoyed frozen (great in smoothies) or in dried form as a tasty snack.

Citrus Fruits

Oranges, clementines, grapefruit, lemons, limes... these juicy fruits are great providers of vitamin C and soluble fiber. We like grapefruit to start the day and oranges as a snack since they travel well.

According to the Scientific Report of the 2015 Dietary Guidelines Advisory Committee, underconsumption of these nutrients in the American diet pose the largest public health threat:

- vitamin D
- calcium
- iron
- potassium
- fiber

Additional nutrients that Americans underconsume include vitamins A, C, and E, as well as folate and magnesium.

You'll also see that many of our recipes call for citrus juices because just a few teaspoons can add the perfect pop of flavor.

Cruciferous Veggies

This variety of nutrient-dense veggies includes cauliflower, broccoli, Brussels sprouts, cabbage, bok choy, and more. Cruciferous veggies are rich in fiber, phytochemicals, vitamins, and minerals. What are phytochemicals, you ask? They are chemical compounds found in plants that are not vitamins and minerals but have been associated with positive effects on health, such as reduced risk for cancer and heart disease.

Get creative with these veggies and incorporate them into a plate of crudités at your next gathering. Or lightly sauté, roast, or steam them as a side at dinner—it's all delicious! You'll see we've used them creatively throughout this book, and we suggest looking in the side dish section for some particularly delicious recipes featuring cruciferous veggies.

Dark Leafy Greens

Spinach, collards, kale, romaine lettuce, mustard greens, watercress, and swiss chard...these nutrient powerhouses provide vitamin C, fiber, folic acid, potassium, magnesium, and iron. They are also very low in carbohydrate so the headline here is to *eat more*! Pair them with other superfoods to create delicious salads, sandwiches, pasta dishes, omelets, or soups.

Fish High in Omega-3 Fatty Acids

We love fish as a healthy protein option, and the American Diabetes Association recommends that most people eat fish at least two to three times per week. Some fish are packed with nutrients called omega-3 fatty acids, which play a role in heart and brain health.

Fish and seafood high in omega-3 fatty acids include salmon, trout, sardines, anchovies, herring, Pacific oysters, and Atlantic and Pacific mackerel. In addition to healthy fats, fish also provide vitamin D and calcium.

Healthy Fats

Diabetes nutrition guidelines have shifted away from promoting a low-fat diet in recent years. Newer research shows that when planning meals for diabetes, it is more important to look at the *type of fat* you're eating rather than the *total amount of fat*.

Healthy fats are the ones to focus on; they may help with blood glucose management and lower the risk of heart disease. Within the healthy fats category, you'll find monounsaturated and polyunsaturated fats. Sources of these healthy fats include most plant-based oils (olive, canola, corn, etc.), avocados, olives, nuts, nut butters, and seeds. Healthy fats are a great tool in the kitchen for cooking other foods and adding flavor.

Can I eat as much healthy fat as I want? While total fat is no longer a main focus when meal planning, it's still important to be mindful of portions when eating healthy fats. All fats—the healthy kind and the less healthy kind—are dense in calories.

Use olive oil when sautéing or roasting veggies or to make homemade salad dressing. Snack on some avocado on toast or dice it up and enjoy it atop a salad or bowl of chili. Nuts, nut butters, and seeds are also little nutrition dynamos—they're great for snacking, adding to salads, spreading on sandwiches, and more!

Herbs and Spices

Pack an extra flavor punch into your meals by getting creative with herbs and spices. While there is still a body of evidence building about the benefits of various herbs and spices, many of these plant-based ingredients have been associated with health benefits. Not to mention, they don't add any extra calories, carbs, or sodium to your dishes. So these are one of THE BEST ways to flavor your food!

Lean Protein

Lean fish, shellfish, eggs (especially the egg whites), and poultry without the skin fall into this category. You may be surprised to see lean protein on our list, but here's our thinking—these foods are high in protein and contain little fat and no carbohydrate. Protein has less of an effect on blood glucose levels, so unless you follow a vegetarian eating pattern, it's a great idea to incorporate these foods into your meals in portions that fit your meal plan.

Legumes—Beans, Peas, and Lentils

These budget-friendly, plant-based proteins are a great choice at mealtime! Legumes also include bean-based foods like hummus, edamame, and soy products. For 1/2 cup of beans, keep in mind that you get about 15–20 grams of carbohydrate, but you also meet approximately 1/3 of your daily fiber needs. When you eat beans, you will also enjoy a boost of magnesium, folate, potassium, and iron.

We never get bored of experimenting with the many types of legumes! Just pick from the plethora of legume options and try them in soups, salads, grain bowls, pasta dishes, wraps, or pretty much anything else. To save time and money, you can look for canned varieties in the store. Just make sure to drain and rinse them before using to keep sodium in check or opt for reduced-sodium varieties.

Low-Fat Milk and Yogurt

Milk and yogurt provide important nutrients such as calcium and protein. These foods also are usually fortified with vitamin D—an extra bonus. When it comes to milk, we opt for nonfat milk whenever possible. And for yogurt, we always compare nutrition information on labels in the yogurt aisle to determine the best pick. Be sure to check on those total carbohydrates if you are counting carbs with diabetes!

We're big fans of the very versatile nonfat, plain Greek yogurt, which you'll see used in a variety of ways throughout this book. It's a protein-packed, lower-carbohydrate option that's great in savory or sweet dishes.

Sweet Potatoes

Sweet potatoes are what we like to call "nature's candy." They are packed with vitamin A, vitamin C, and potassium. They also have a lower glycemic index than regular potatoes, so they won't raise your blood glucose as much. They are a starchy vegetable, so it's important to eat them in proper portions—1/2 cup cooked has about 15 grams of carbohydrate.

Tomatoes

Tomatoes—a tasty nonstarchy vegetable option that's packed with nutrients including vitamins A, C and E, as well as potassium. They also are high in lycopene, an antioxidant that has been linked to many health benefits.

Whole Grains

Whole grains include oats, whole wheat, barley, brown rice, quinoa, farro, and even popcorn. Try to make at least half of the grains you eat whole grains—if not more! It's a simple swap from white rice to brown rice or from white bread to a more nutty, flavorful wheat bread. Whole grains provide dietary fiber and have been linked to heart health, which is important for people with diabetes because of their increased risk of heart disease. Whole grains also offer a host of vitamins and minerals.

Whole grains are the stars of many recipes within this book. We love experimenting in the kitchen with all sorts of grains to create tasty cereals, grain bowls, soups, and more.

SUPERFOOD SWAPS - TRY THEM OUT!

Instead of...	Try...
Sour cream	Nonfat, plain Greek yogurt
Butter or lard	Oils in cooking
Fatty cuts of meat	Fish or another lean protein (turkey, chicken without the skin)
White bread and other refined grains	Whole-grain foods such as 100% whole-wheat bread, brown rice, quinoa
Full-fat milk or yogurt	Low-fat milk or yogurt
Potato chips and dip at snack time	100% whole-wheat pita or veggies with hummus
Added sugar to sweeten foods	Dried fruit
Sweetened yogurt	Plain yogurt flavored with fruit and nuts
Cheese on your sandwich or burger	Tomato and avocado

The Fruit and Veggie Caveat

It's no secret that American diets are lacking fruits and vegetables. Yet, they are the best "bang for our buck" when it comes to nutrition. For this reason, we think it's important to recognize that while we've called out a few specific varieties above, all fruits and vegetables truly are superfoods.

Regardless of type, fruits and vegetables provide us with essential vitamins, minerals, and fiber. So, don't let our list above leave you feeling limited. We highly encourage you to generally focus on including more of these foods as your meal plan allows!

SUPERFOOD-INSPIRED RECIPES

Breakfast

Cauliflower Hash Browns

Look no further for a great, lower-carb breakfast alternative to fried potatoes.

INGREDIENTS

1/2 small head cauliflower
1 bunch green onions (about 1/4 cup)
1 Tbsp olive oil
1/4 tsp garlic powder
1/4 tsp coarse black pepper
1/16 tsp salt

Prep Time: 10 minutes
Cook Time: 20 minutes
Serves: 2
Serving Size: 3/4 cup

DIRECTIONS

1. Place raw cauliflower in a food processor, and process into rice-size pieces (this should yield about 1 1/2 cups). Set aside.
2. In a large pan, sauté green onions in olive oil for about 5 minutes.
3. Add cauliflower and sauté for about 15 minutes over medium-low heat until pieces soften.
4. Sprinkle with garlic powder, pepper, and salt.

Tip: Serve with Fried Egg with Spinach (page 5). If short on time, use packaged riced cauliflower.

BASIC NUTRITIONAL VALUES

Calories	90
Calories from Fat	60
Total Fat	**7.0 g**
Saturated Fat	1.1 g
Trans Fat	0.0 g
Cholesterol	**0 mg**
Sodium	**100 mg**
Potassium	**330 mg**
Total Carbohydrate	**6 g**
Dietary Fiber	2 g
Sugars	2 g
Protein	**2 g**
Phosphorus	**50 mg**

CHOICES/EXCHANGES

1 Nonstarchy Vegetable, 1 1/2 Fat

Fried Egg with Spinach

Try sautéing leftover greens for a savory addition to breakfast dishes.

INGREDIENTS

1/2 cup chopped onion
1 tsp olive oil
3 cups fresh spinach
2 eggs

DIRECTIONS

1. In a skillet, sauté onions in olive oil for about 5 minutes.
2. Add fresh spinach to the skillet and sauté about 3 minutes.
3. In the skillet, divide the spinach mixture into 2 fairly flat sections.
4. Crack one egg over each spinach section and cook for 5 minutes. Flip and continue cooking until cooked through.*

*Eggs should be cooked until both the white and yolk are firm.

Tip: Serve with Cauliflower Hash Browns (page 4).

Prep Time: 5 minutes
Cook Time: 15 minutes
Serves: 2
Serving Size: 1 egg with 1/4 cup cooked spinach

BASIC NUTRITIONAL VALUES

Calories	**120**
Calories from Fat	60
Total Fat	**7.0 g**
Saturated Fat	1.9 g
Trans Fat	0.0 g
Cholesterol	**185 mg**
Sodium	**110 mg**
Potassium	**380 mg**
Total Carbohydrate	**6 g**
Dietary Fiber	2 g
Sugars	2 g
Protein	**8 g**
Phosphorus	**135 mg**

CHOICES/EXCHANGES

1 Nonstarchy Vegetable,
1 Medium-Fat Protein, 1/2 Fat

Mini Red Pepper and Mushroom Frittatas

These mini frittatas make a delicious breakfast. Enjoy them fresh out of the oven on the weekend or for breakfast over the next few days. Just store them in the refrigerator (in a tightly sealed container) and heat them up in the morning for a quick breakfast!

INGREDIENTS

Nonstick cooking spray
3 strips turkey bacon
1 1/2 tsp olive oil
1 red pepper, finely diced
2 cups sliced mushrooms
1/2 cup finely diced onion
5 eggs
1/2 cup nonfat milk
1/2 cup shredded pepper jack cheese
Freshly ground black pepper

Prep Time: 25 minutes
Cook Time: 20 minutes
Serves: 10
Serving Size: 1 mini frittata

DIRECTIONS

1. Spray 10 muffin cups in a muffin pan with cooking spray and preheat oven to 375°F.
2. In a large nonstick sauté pan, cook turkey bacon until done.
3. Remove turkey bacon from pan and dice, then set aside. Add olive oil, red pepper, mushrooms, and onion to the hot sauté pan and cook, stirring occasionally, until cooked through. Then remove from heat.
4. While veggies are cooking, whisk together 5 eggs, milk, cheese, and pepper.
5. Pour egg mixture evenly into 10 muffin cups (each cup should be about 2/3 full) and spoon veggie mixture and bacon into each cup to fill it.
6. Bake in the oven for 20 minutes.

BASIC NUTRITIONAL VALUES

Calories	**90**
Calories from Fat	50
Total Fat	**6.0 g**
Saturated Fat	2.1 g
Trans Fat	0.0 g
Cholesterol	**100 mg**
Sodium	**115 mg**
Potassium	**160 mg**
Total Carbohydrate	**3 g**
Dietary Fiber	1 g
Sugars	2 g
Protein	**6 g**
Phosphorus	**125 mg**

CHOICES/EXCHANGES

1 Medium-Fat Protein

Oatmeal Pecan Pancakes

Finely chopped oats can make an easy, whole-grain alternative to wheat flour in many recipes such as these pancakes. Serve these with the Blueberry Sauce on page 29.

INGREDIENTS

1 cup quick oats
1 1/2 tsp baking powder
2 eggs
1/3 cup nonfat milk
1/3 cup mashed banana (about 1/2 medium banana)
1/2 tsp vanilla
2 Tbsp chopped pecans
1 Tbsp canola oil

Prep Time: 10 minutes
Cook Time: 15 minutes
Serves: 6
Serving Size: 1 pancake

DIRECTIONS

1. Using a food processor, process the oats to a flour-like consistency. Mix oats and baking powder in a small bowl and set aside.
2. In a separate bowl, mix eggs, milk, mashed banana, and vanilla. Add to dry ingredients.
3. Stir in pecans.
4. Heat oil in nonstick skillet over medium heat.
5. Drop 1/4 cup of batter onto the hot skillet to make each pancake. Cook until lightly brown on both sides.

BASIC NUTRITIONAL VALUES

Calories	130
Calories from Fat	60
Total Fat	**7.0 g**
Saturated Fat	1.0 g
Trans Fat	0.0 g
Cholesterol	**60 mg**
Sodium	**120 mg**
Potassium	**150 mg**
Total Carbohydrate	**13 g**
Dietary Fiber	2 g
Sugars	3 g
Protein	**5 g**
Phosphorus	**225 mg**

CHOICES/EXCHANGES

1 Starch, 1 Fat

On-the-Go PB&J Oatmeal

This recipe makes for a perfect breakfast at the office—all you need is access to a microwave. To bring this oatmeal on-the-go, pack your oats and cinnamon in one container and golden raisins and peanut butter in another. Put it all together once you get to the office.

INGREDIENTS

1/3 cup old-fashioned oats
1/4 tsp cinnamon
2/3 cup water
1 Tbsp golden raisins
1 Tbsp peanut butter

Prep Time: 2 minutes
Cook Time: 1 minute
Serves: 1
Serving Size: About 2/3 cup

DIRECTIONS

1. In a large cereal bowl, stir together old-fashioned oats and cinnamon. Add water and microwave for 1 minute and 15 seconds, or until oatmeal is cooked. (Cook time may vary by microwave.)
2. Remove oats from the microwave and mix in raisins and peanut butter.

BASIC NUTRITIONAL VALUES

Calories	**220**
Calories from Fat	90
Total Fat	**10.0 g**
Saturated Fat	2.0 g
Trans Fat	0.0 g
Cholesterol	**0 mg**
Sodium	**75 mg**
Potassium	**270 mg**
Total Carbohydrate	**29 g**
Dietary Fiber	4 g
Sugars	7 g
Protein	**8 g**
Phosphorus	**180 mg**

CHOICES/EXCHANGES

1 1/2 Starch, 1/2 Fruit,
1 High-Fat Protein

Open-Faced Egg Sandwiches

Forget the drive-thru! This egg sandwich is just as juicy and delicious as a fast-food breakfast, while packing in extra nutrients.

INGREDIENTS

Nonstick cooking spray
4 (1/2-inch) beefsteak or heirloom tomato slices
1/2 tsp dried basil
1/2 tsp freshly ground black pepper
1/8 tsp salt
2 eggs
1 whole-wheat English muffin, sliced in half
2 Tbsp shredded sharp cheddar cheese
1 cup arugula

Prep Time: 10 minutes
Cook Time: 5 minutes
Serves: 2
Serving Size: 1 open-faced sandwich

DIRECTIONS

1. Preheat oven to 400°F (or set a toaster oven at 400°F).
2. Cover a small baking pan with foil and lightly coat with cooking spray. Place tomato slices on foil and sprinkle with dried basil, pepper, and salt. Lightly spray tops of tomatoes with cooking spray and place in the oven to roast for 10 minutes.
3. While tomatoes are cooking, heat a large frying pan coated lightly with cooking spray over medium-high heat. Whisk eggs in a small bowl. Once pan is hot, add eggs and cook until scrambled. Turn off heat. Sprinkle cheese over the eggs, and allow to melt for another 30 seconds.
4. Place half of the egg mixture on 1/2 of the English muffin and top with 1/2 cup arugula. Repeat with the remaining egg mixture, 1/2 English muffin, and arugula. Then, remove tomatoes from oven and top each open-faced sandwich with two tomato slices.

BASIC NUTRITIONAL VALUES

Calories	**180**
Calories from Fat	70
Total Fat	**8.0 g**
Saturated Fat	3.2 g
Trans Fat	0.1 g
Cholesterol	**195 mg**
Sodium	**420 mg**
Potassium	**330 mg**
Total Carbohydrate	**17 g**
Dietary Fiber	3 g
Sugars	5 g
Protein	**12 g**
Phosphorus	**250 mg**

CHOICES/EXCHANGES

1 Starch, 1 Nonstarchy Vegetable, 1 Medium-Fat Protein

Parmesan Grits

Grits come alive with the addition of herbs and spices—no butter needed!

INGREDIENTS

1 1/2 cups water
1/2 cup corn grits
3 Tbsp chopped green onion
2 cloves garlic, chopped
1/2 tsp olive oil
1 1/2 Tbsp freshly grated Parmesan cheese
1/2 tsp dried thyme
1/4 tsp freshly ground black pepper
1/8 tsp ground sage
1/8 tsp salt

DIRECTIONS

1. Heat water to a boil in a small saucepan and add grits. Reduce heat to low and cook about 5 minutes, stirring continuously.
2. In a small sauté pan, sauté onion and garlic in olive oil for about 3 minutes.
3. Add onions and garlic to grits.
4. Add the rest of the ingredients to grits and mix.

Prep Time: 5 minutes
Cook Time: 10 minutes
Serves: 5
Serving Size: 1/3 cup

BASIC NUTRITIONAL VALUES

Calories	60
Calories from Fat	10
Total Fat	**1.0 g**
Saturated Fat	0.3 g
Trans Fat	0.0 g
Cholesterol	**0 mg**
Sodium	**80 mg**
Potassium	**40 mg**
Total Carbohydrate	**12 g**
Dietary Fiber	1 g
Sugars	0 g
Protein	**2 g**
Phosphorus	**25 mg**

CHOICES/EXCHANGES

1 Starch

Pumpkin Flaxseed Pancakes

Almond flour adds a subtle sweet taste to dishes and is a great alternative to wheat flour for lower-carbohydrate baked goods.

INGREDIENTS

1/2 cup quick oats, ground to a flour-like consistency
1 cup almond flour
1 1/2 tsp baking powder
1/2 tsp nutmeg
1 tsp cinnamon
4 eggs
1/2 cup unsweetened vanilla almond milk
1 cup pumpkin purée
1 tsp vanilla
1 Tbsp flaxseeds
2 Tbsp canola oil

Prep Time: 10 minutes
Cook Time: 15 minutes
Serves: 6
Serving Size: 2 pancakes

DIRECTIONS

1. In a large bowl, mix oats, almond flour, baking powder, nutmeg, and cinnamon together and set aside.
2. In a separate bowl, mix eggs, almond milk, pumpkin, and vanilla. Add to dry ingredients. Stir in flaxseeds.
3. Heat oil in a nonstick skillet over medium heat.
4. Drop 1/4 cup of batter onto the hot skillet to make each pancake. If batter is thick, flatten it to decrease cooking time.
5. Cook until lightly brown on each side (about 3–4 minutes on each side).

BASIC NUTRITIONAL VALUES

Calories	**250**
Calories from Fat	170
Total Fat	**19.0 g**
Saturated Fat	2.4 g
Trans Fat	0.0 g
Cholesterol	**125 mg**
Sodium	**160 mg**
Potassium	**320 mg**
Total Carbohydrate	**13 g**
Dietary Fiber	5 g
Sugars	3 g
Protein	**10 g**
Phosphorus	**325 mg**

CHOICES/EXCHANGES

1 Starch, 1 Medium-Fat Protein, 2 1/2 Fat

Pumpkin Overnight Oats

Make this the night before and you can enjoy it for breakfast over the next several days. Eat overnight oats cold, or warm them up in the microwave—whatever suits your taste!

INGREDIENTS

1 cup plain soy milk
1/2 cup pumpkin purée
1/2 tsp cinnamon
1/4 tsp nutmeg
1 Tbsp honey
1 cup old-fashioned oats
4 Tbsp chopped roasted pecans, divided

Prep Time: 10 minutes
Refrigeration Time: Overnight
Cook Time: N/A
Serves: 4
Serving Size: 1/2 cup oats and 1 Tbsp chopped pecans

DIRECTIONS

1. In a medium mixing bowl, whisk together soy milk, pumpkin, cinnamon, nutmeg, and honey until thoroughly mixed.
2. Stir in the oats, cover with a tight-fitting lid or plastic wrap, and refrigerate overnight.
3. To serve, sprinkle 1 Tbsp chopped pecans over each 1/2 cup of oats.

Tip: Keep your morning routine quick and easy! Store 1/2 cup portions of these overnight oats in separate containers to easily "grab-and-go" in the morning.

BASIC NUTRITIONAL VALUES

Calories	**180**
Calories from Fat	70
Total Fat	**8.0 g**
Saturated Fat	0.9 g
Trans Fat	0.0 g
Cholesterol	**0 mg**
Sodium	**30 mg**
Potassium	**260 mg**
Total Carbohydrate	**24 g**
Dietary Fiber	4 g
Sugars	7 g
Protein	**6 g**
Phosphorus	**145 mg**

CHOICES/EXCHANGES

1 1/2 Starch, 1 1/2 Fat

Savory Quinoa Breakfast Bowls

This flavor-filled dish will make you think you're out on the town for brunch.

INGREDIENTS

Nonstick cooking spray
2 eggs
1 cup warm, cooked quinoa
1 1/2 cups arugula
1 cup Garlic-Thyme Roasted Mushrooms and Carrots (page 142)
3 tsp crumbled goat cheese
Freshly ground black pepper, to taste

Prep Time: 5 minutes
Cook Time: 5 minutes
Serves: 2
Serving Size: 1 quinoa bowl

DIRECTIONS

1. Spray skillet well with cooking spray and heat over medium heat.
2. Crack both eggs into the skillet and cook 1–2 minutes per side or until both the white and yolk are firm.
3. To assemble one quinoa bowl, place 1/2 cup quinoa in the bottom of an individual serving bowl and top with 3/4 cup arugula, 1 cooked egg, 1/2 cup Garlic-Thyme Roasted Mushrooms and Carrots, and 1 1/2 tsp goat cheese. Repeat to assemble second quinoa bowl. Top both quinoa bowls with freshly ground pepper to taste.

BASIC NUTRITIONAL VALUES

Calories	**270**
Calories from Fat	100
Total Fat	**11.0 g**
Saturated Fat	2.9 g
Trans Fat	0.0 g
Cholesterol	**190 mg**
Sodium	**150 mg**
Potassium	**660 mg**
Total Carbohydrate	**30 g**
Dietary Fiber	5 g
Sugars	7 g
Protein	**13 g**
Phosphorus	**320 mg**

CHOICES/EXCHANGES

1 1/2 Starch, 2 Nonstarchy Vegetable, 1 Medium-Fat Protein, 1/2 Fat

Southwest Tofu Scramble

This scramble makes for a delicious savory breakfast, but you can also enjoy it for lunch or dinner as a vegetarian option that is chock full of superfoods like tomatoes, black beans, and more!

INGREDIENTS

1/4 tsp smoked paprika
1/2 tsp garlic powder
2 tsp cumin
1/4 tsp freshly ground black pepper
1/4 tsp salt
2 tsp olive oil
14 oz extra-firm tofu, drained well and mashed with a fork
1 Tbsp finely diced jalapeño pepper (seeds and ribs removed)
1 cup diced tomatoes
1 (15-oz) can reduced-sodium black beans, drained and rinsed
1/4 cup shredded reduced-fat sharp cheddar cheese

Prep Time: 10 minutes
Cook Time: 12 minutes
Serves: 4
Serving Size: 1 cup

DIRECTIONS

1. In a small bowl, combine paprika, garlic powder, cumin, pepper, and salt. Set aside.
2. In a large nonstick skillet, heat olive oil over medium heat. Add tofu and jalapeño and cook for 5 minutes, stirring occasionally. Add tomatoes and spice mixture and cook another 5 minutes, stirring occasionally.
3. Add black beans and cook until heated through.
4. Remove pan from heat and sprinkle cheese over top.
5. Serve hot. If you like extra spice, add a little hot sauce to each 1-cup portion of scramble (optional).

BASIC NUTRITIONAL VALUES

Calories	230
Calories from Fat	80
Total Fat	**9.0 g**
Saturated Fat	1.9 g
Trans Fat	0.0 g
Cholesterol	**9 mg**
Sodium	**330 mg**
Potassium	**500 mg**
Total Carbohydrate	**21 g**
Dietary Fiber	7 g
Sugars	2 g
Protein	**18 g**
Phosphorus	**275 mg**

CHOICES/EXCHANGES

1 1/2 Starch, 2 Medium-Fat Protein

Zucchini Quinoa Fritters with Feta

These are fun for breakfast or a snack, and they're a great way to slip more nonstarchy veggies into your day.

INGREDIENTS

3/4 cup shredded zucchini
1 egg
1/4 cup cooked quinoa
1/4 tsp freshly ground black pepper
1/4 cup finely diced onion
1 clove garlic, minced
1/2 tsp olive oil
1 tomato, chopped
2 Tbsp crumbled feta cheese

Prep Time: 15 minutes
Cook Time: 10 minutes
Serves: 5
Serving Size: 2 fritters

DIRECTIONS

1. Squeeze out all the liquid from the shredded zucchini between paper towels. Let sit while combining other ingredients.
2. In a mixing bowl, mix egg, quinoa, and pepper together and set aside.
3. In a nonstick skillet, sauté onion and garlic in olive oil.
4. Mix the zucchini, onion, and garlic together with the egg and quinoa mixture in the mixing bowl.
5. Drop mixture by spoonful onto hot skillet, making 10 fritters.
6. Cook on both sides over medium-high heat until golden brown.
7. Top with chopped tomato and crumbled feta.

BASIC NUTRITIONAL VALUES

Calories	**50**
Calories from Fat	20
Total Fat	**2.5 g**
Saturated Fat	1.0 g
Trans Fat	0.0 g
Cholesterol	**40 mg**
Sodium	**60 mg**
Potassium	**180 mg**
Total Carbohydrate	**5 g**
Dietary Fiber	1 g
Sugars	2 g
Protein	**3 g**
Phosphorus	**65 mg**

CHOICES/EXCHANGES

1 Nonstarchy Vegetable,
1/2 Fat

Breakfast Pepper Sauté

Peppers get sweeter while cooking, creating a sweet and savory mix of flavors. Try serving the sauté with Parmesan Grits (page 10) for a hearty breakfast. This is also a great dish to serve over rice for dinner.

INGREDIENTS

2 sweet peppers (we used red and yellow), cut into small pieces (about 2 cups)
1 cup chopped red onion
2 cloves garlic, finely chopped
2 tsp olive oil
2 cooked garlic chicken sausage links (about 2.4 oz each), cut into small pieces

Prep Time: 10 minutes
Cook Time: 30 minutes
Serves: 4
Serving Size: 1/2 cup pepper mix

DIRECTIONS

1. In a nonstick skillet over medium-high heat, sauté peppers, onion, and garlic in olive oil for about 10 minutes or until soft.
2. Add sausage pieces to skillet. Cooking until warmed through, flipping to brown on both sides (about 5 minutes).

BASIC NUTRITIONAL VALUES

Calories	**120**
Calories from Fat	45
Total Fat	**5.0 g**
Saturated Fat	0.5 g
Trans Fat	0.0 g
Cholesterol	**25 mg**
Sodium	**200 mg**
Potassium	**450 mg**
Total Carbohydrate	**11 g**
Dietary Fiber	2 g
Sugars	4 g
Protein	**7 g**
Phosphorus	**110 mg**

CHOICES/EXCHANGES

2 Nonstarchy Vegetable,
1 Lean Protein, 1/2 Fat

Breakfast Tacos

Tortillas are a great quick breakfast ingredient. Try filling them with eggs or leftover protein from dinner.

INGREDIENTS

1/3 cup chopped green onions
1/2 tsp olive oil
2 whole eggs plus 2 egg whites
2 Tbsp nonfat milk
1/4 cup canned black beans, drained and rinsed
1/4 cup salsa
2 Tbsp mashed avocado
6 (6-inch) corn tortillas

Prep Time: 10 minutes
Cook Time: 10 minutes
Serves: 3
Serving Size: 2 tacos

DIRECTIONS

1. In a nonstick skillet, sauté onion in olive oil over medium heat for about 5 minutes.
2. In a mixing bowl, whisk eggs and whites together with milk.
3. Add egg mixture to skillet with onion and cook until cooked through (about 5 minutes).
4. Add black beans to skillet to warm.
5. In a small bowl, mix salsa and mashed avocado together to make topping.
6. Top each tortilla with 1/4 cup egg/bean mixture and 1 Tbsp topping. Serve warm.

Tip: We recommend serving with 1/2 cup fresh sliced strawberries on the side for a colorful, balanced breakfast.

BASIC NUTRITIONAL VALUES

Calories	**230**
Calories from Fat	60
Total Fat	**7.0 g**
Saturated Fat	1.6 g
Trans Fat	0.0 g
Cholesterol	**125 mg**
Sodium	**240 mg**
Potassium	**370 mg**
Total Carbohydrate	**31 g**
Dietary Fiber	5 g
Sugars	3 g
Protein	**12 g**
Phosphorus	**280 mg**

CHOICES/EXCHANGES

2 Starch, 1 Medium-Fat
Protein

Dressings, Sauces, and Marinades

Homemade Balsamic Dressing

Make your own salad dressing at home and you can eliminate a lot of the sodium and other additives that are found in store-bought dressings.

INGREDIENTS

1/2 cup balsamic vinegar
1/4 cup olive oil
1 tsp Dijon mustard
1/2 tsp freshly ground black pepper

Prep Time: 5 minutes
Cook Time: N/A
Serves: 6
Serving Size: 2 Tbsp

DIRECTIONS

1. In a small bowl, whisk all dressing ingredients together until combined.

BASIC NUTRITIONAL VALUES

Calories	**100**
Calories from Fat	80
Total Fat	**9.0 g**
Saturated Fat	1.2 g
Trans Fat	0.0 g
Cholesterol	**0 mg**
Sodium	**25 mg**
Potassium	**25 mg**
Total Carbohydrate	**4 g**
Dietary Fiber	0 g
Sugars	3 g
Protein	**0 g**
Phosphorus	**5 mg**

CHOICES/EXCHANGES

2 Fat

Pesto Vinaigrette

This pesto vinaigrette makes a great marinade for fish or chicken. You can also use it as a dressing to make veggies or salads pop. Try it in our recipe Tilapia with Pesto Vinaigrette and Tomatoes (page 106).

INGREDIENTS

2 Tbsp store-bought pesto
1/4 cup plus 2 Tbsp red wine vinegar
2 Tbsp olive oil
1 shallot, finely diced
Freshly ground black pepper, to taste

Prep Time: 5 minutes
Cook Time: N/A
Serves: 5
Serving Size: 2 Tbsp

DIRECTIONS

1. In a small bowl or dressing container, mix all dressing ingredients together until combined.

> **Tip:** If you have time, allow the dressing to sit for at least 1 hour before using so the shallot marinates and absorbs the dressing flavors.

BASIC NUTRITIONAL VALUES

Calories	70
Calories from Fat	60
Total Fat	**7.0 g**
Saturated Fat	1.0 g
Trans Fat	0.0 g
Cholesterol	**0 mg**
Sodium	**70 mg**
Potassium	**25 mg**
Total Carbohydrate	**1 g**
Dietary Fiber	0 g
Sugars	0 g
Protein	**0 g**
Phosphorus	**5 mg**

CHOICES/EXCHANGES

1 1/2 Fat

Rosemary Honey Mustard Dipping Sauce

Flavorful, sweet, and slightly tangy, this dipping sauce pairs well with our Sweet Potato Fries (page 83).

INGREDIENTS

1/4 cup nonfat, plain Greek yogurt
1 1/2 tsp spicy mustard
1/2 tsp honey
1 tsp dried rosemary leaves, crushed

Prep Time: 10 minutes
Cook Time: N/A
Serves: 5
Serving Size: 1 Tbsp

DIRECTIONS

1. In a small bowl, mix all ingredients together until combined. This dressing can be made ahead of time and kept refrigerated for up to a week.

BASIC NUTRITIONAL VALUES

Calories	10
Calories from Fat	0
Total Fat	**0.0 g**
Saturated Fat	0.0 g
Trans Fat	0.0 g
Cholesterol	**0 mg**
Sodium	**20 mg**
Potassium	**20 mg**
Total Carbohydrate	**1 g**
Dietary Fiber	0 g
Sugars	1 g
Protein	**1 g**
Phosphorus	**15 mg**

CHOICES/EXCHANGES

Free food

Spicy Peanut Dressing

This spicy dressing is used in the Spicy Peanut Broccoli Slaw recipe (page 52) and can also be used as a dipping sauce, marinade, or stir-fry sauce.

INGREDIENTS

3 Tbsp water
1/4 cup powdered peanut butter
1 Tbsp rice wine vinegar
1 1/2 tsp reduced-sodium soy sauce
1/2 tsp honey
1 Tbsp finely chopped fresh ginger
1/4 tsp red pepper flakes (use less if you do not like spicy)

Prep Time: 5 minutes
Cook Time: N/A
Serves: 6
Serving Size: 1 1/2 Tbsp

DIRECTIONS

1. In a small bowl, mix water and peanut butter powder together.
2. Add remaining dressing ingredients and mix well.

BASIC NUTRITIONAL VALUES

Calories	20
Calories from Fat	5
Total Fat	**0.5 g**
Saturated Fat	0.1 g
Trans Fat	0.0 g
Cholesterol	**0 mg**
Sodium	**75 mg**
Potassium	**55 mg**
Total Carbohydrate	**3 g**
Dietary Fiber	1 g
Sugars	1 g
Protein	**2 g**
Phosphorus	**25 mg**

CHOICES/EXCHANGES

Free food

Strawberry Maple Topping

This is a quick superfood topping for yogurt or to try on Pumpkin Pancakes (page 11).

INGREDIENTS

8 oz strawberries, sliced
2 tsp maple syrup
2 Tbsp water

Prep Time: 5 minutes
Cook Time: N/A
Serves: 8
Serving Size: 2 Tbsp

DIRECTIONS

1. Place all ingredients in a blender and blend until desired texture is reached.

BASIC NUTRITIONAL VALUES	
Calories	15
Calories from Fat	0
Total Fat	**0.0 g**
Saturated Fat	0.0 g
Trans Fat	0.0 g
Cholesterol	**0 mg**
Sodium	**0 mg**
Potassium	**45 mg**
Total Carbohydrate	**3 g**
Dietary Fiber	1 g
Sugars	2 g
Protein	**0 g**
Phosphorus	**5 mg**

CHOICES/EXCHANGES

Free food

Tahini Sauce

Try this tasty sauce on almost any wrap or sandwich. We especially like it on our Edamame Veggie Wrap (page 44)!

INGREDIENTS

1/3 cup tahini
1/4 cup lemon juice
2 cloves garlic
3 Tbsp water
Freshly ground black pepper, to taste

Prep Time: 5 minutes
Cook Time: N/A
Serves: 6
Serving Size: 2 Tbsp

DIRECTIONS

1. Add all ingredients to a small food processor or blender. Blend until smooth.

BASIC NUTRITIONAL VALUES

Calories	60
Calories from Fat	45
Total Fat	**5.0 g**
Saturated Fat	0.8 g
Trans Fat	0.0 g
Cholesterol	**0 mg**
Sodium	**15 mg**
Potassium	**55 mg**
Total Carbohydrate	**3 g**
Dietary Fiber	1 g
Sugars	0 g
Protein	**2 g**
Phosphorus	**75 mg**

CHOICES/EXCHANGES

1 Fat

White Balsamic, Orange, and Chia Seed Dressing

This dressing uses fruit juice for a light, sweet-tasting salad dressing. Serve with Mixed Greens with Spicy Pecans, Goat Cheese, and Pear (page 48).

INGREDIENTS

2 Tbsp plus 2 tsp fresh orange juice
1 tsp white balsamic vinegar
1 Tbsp olive oil
1/4 tsp chia seeds
1/8 tsp white pepper
1/8 tsp cinnamon

Prep Time: 10 minutes
Cook Time: N/A
Serves: 4
Serving Size: 1 Tbsp

DIRECTIONS

1. In a small bowl, mix all dressing ingredients together until combined.

BASIC NUTRITIONAL VALUES

Calories	35
Calories from Fat	30
Total Fat	**3.5 g**
Saturated Fat	0.5 g
Trans Fat	0.0 g
Cholesterol	**0 mg**
Sodium	**0 mg**
Potassium	**25 mg**
Total Carbohydrate	**2 g**
Dietary Fiber	0 g
Sugars	1 g
Protein	**0 g**
Phosphorus	**5 mg**

CHOICES/EXCHANGES

1 Fat

White Balsamic Vinaigrette

This flavor-filled salad dressing will make any salad "pop." We especially like it with our Spinach, Avocado, and Summer Berry Salad (page 53) or our Mixed Greens with Strawberries, Feta, and Turkey Bacon salad (page 49).

INGREDIENTS

2 Tbsp olive oil
2 Tbsp white balsamic vinegar
1 tsp honey
1/2 large lime, juiced
1 clove garlic, minced
1/4 tsp freshly ground black pepper

Prep Time: 5 minutes
Cook Time: N/A
Serves: 6
Serving Size: 1 Tbsp

DIRECTIONS

1. In a small bowl, whisk all dressing ingredients together until combined. Store in a tightly sealed container or dressing carafe in the refrigerator.

Tip: Keep it on hand! You can easily double or triple this recipe to make additional dressing so you'll have plenty on hand at mealtime.

BASIC NUTRITIONAL VALUES

Calories	50
Calories from Fat	40
Total Fat	**4.5 g**
Saturated Fat	0.6 g
Trans Fat	0.0 g
Cholesterol	**0 mg**
Sodium	**0 mg**
Potassium	**15 mg**
Total Carbohydrate	**3 g**
Dietary Fiber	0 g
Sugars	2 g
Protein	**0 g**
Phosphorus	**0 mg**

CHOICES/EXCHANGES

1 Fat

Avocado Cilantro Dressing

This dressing comes together easily with the help of a small food processor or blender. Enjoy it drizzled over our Black Bean Quinoa Cakes over Mixed Greens (page 56), or try it over any other salad!

INGREDIENTS

1 small avocado, peeled and pitted
1/2 cup cilantro leaves
2 Tbsp olive oil
2 Tbsp lime juice
1/4 tsp salt
1/2 cup water

Prep Time: 10 minutes
Cook Time: N/A
Serves: 8
Serving Size: 2 Tbsp

DIRECTIONS

1. Add all dressing ingredients to a small food processor or blender. Blend until smooth.

BASIC NUTRITIONAL VALUES

Calories	**50**
Calories from Fat	45
Total Fat	**5.0 g**
Saturated Fat	0.7 g
Trans Fat	0.0 g
Cholesterol	**0 mg**
Sodium	**75 mg**
Potassium	**80 mg**
Total Carbohydrate	**1 g**
Dietary Fiber	1 g
Sugars	0 g
Protein	**0 g**
Phosphorus	**10 mg**

CHOICES/EXCHANGES

1 Fat

Blueberry Sauce

This sauce is packed with flavor and transforms the simplest plain yogurt into a zesty dessert. Use it on Oatmeal Pecan Pancakes (page 7) instead of syrup for a nutrient-packed breakfast.

INGREDIENTS

2 cups fresh blueberries
1 tsp canola oil
Juice of 1 lime (about 2 Tbsp)
1/2 tsp vanilla extract

Prep Time: 5 minutes
Cook Time: 15 minutes
Serves: 6
Serving Size: 2 Tbsp

DIRECTIONS

1. In a nonstick skillet, sauté blueberries in canola oil over low heat for about 10 minutes or until you can crush the berries.
2. Add lime juice and cook another 5 minutes.
3. Remove from heat and stir in vanilla extract.

BASIC NUTRITIONAL VALUES

Calories	**35**
Calories from Fat	10
Total Fat	**1.0 g**
Saturated Fat	0.1 g
Trans Fat	0.0 g
Cholesterol	**0 mg**
Sodium	**0 mg**
Potassium	**40 mg**
Total Carbohydrate	**7 g**
Dietary Fiber	1 g
Sugars	5 g
Protein	**0 g**
Phosphorus	**5 mg**

CHOICES/EXCHANGES

1/2 Fruit

Simple Garlic Marinara Sauce

This marinara sauce is simple to make and can be served with a side of pasta or spaghetti squash, or used in other dishes such as Italian Stuffed Green Peppers (page 120).

INGREDIENTS

4 cloves garlic, crushed
1 tsp olive oil
1 (28-oz) can crushed tomatoes with basil
1/2 cup chopped fresh basil

Prep Time: 5 minutes
Cook Time: 20 minutes
Serves: 6
Serving Size: 1/2 cup

DIRECTIONS

1. In a medium saucepan over low heat, sauté crushed garlic in olive oil.
2. Add tomatoes and basil, and cook on low for at least 20 minutes, stirring often.

BASIC NUTRITIONAL VALUES

Calories	**50**
Calories from Fat	10
Total Fat	**1.0 g**
Saturated Fat	0.2 g
Trans Fat	0.0 g
Cholesterol	**0 mg**
Sodium	**180 mg**
Potassium	**410 mg**
Total Carbohydrate	**10 g**
Dietary Fiber	3 g
Sugars	6 g
Protein	**2 g**
Phosphorus	**50 mg**

CHOICES/EXCHANGES

2 Nonstarchy Vegetable

Greek Yogurt Marinade/Dressing

This marinade is featured in our Greek Yogurt–Marinated Grilled Chicken recipe (page 109), but it can also be used to marinate fish or as a dressing over cooked veggies or salad!

INGREDIENTS

2/3 cup nonfat, plain Greek yogurt
1 Tbsp olive oil
Zest and juice of 1 lemon
1 clove garlic, crushed or minced
1 tsp dried oregano
1/4 tsp red pepper flakes

Prep Time: 5 minutes
Cook Time: N/A
Serves: 6
Serving Size: 2 Tbsp

DIRECTIONS

1. In a small bowl, whisk all ingredients together until combined.

BASIC NUTRITIONAL VALUES

Calories	40
Calories from Fat	20
Total Fat	**2.5 g**
Saturated Fat	0.3 g
Trans Fat	0.0 g
Cholesterol	**0 mg**
Sodium	**10 mg**
Potassium	**50 mg**
Total Carbohydrate	**2 g**
Dietary Fiber	0 g
Sugars	1 g
Protein	**3 g**
Phosphorus	**35 mg**

CHOICES/EXCHANGES

1/2 Fat

Sandwiches, Soups, and Chilis

Mediterranean Chicken Pita

This recipe makes for a simple, delicious sandwich. Enjoy it for lunch or dinner with a salad or another quick vegetable side dish!

INGREDIENTS

2 cups cubed roasted chicken (can use leftover or rotisserie chicken)
1/2 cup low-fat tzatziki sauce (such as Trader Joe's)
2 whole-wheat pitas, cut in half (to make 4 pita pockets)
1 cup diced cucumber
1 cup diced tomato
1/2 cup unsalted, sliced dry-roasted almonds

Prep Time: 10 minutes
Cook Time: N/A
Serves: 4
Serving Size: 1 pita pocket

DIRECTIONS

1. In a medium mixing bowl, mix together chicken and tzatziki sauce. Stuff 1/2 cup of chicken mixture into each pita pocket.
2. Top each filled pita pocket with 1/4 cup cucumbers, 1/4 cup tomatoes, and 2 Tbsp sliced almonds.

Tip: You can always make one pita and save the rest of your ingredients in the refrigerator to use as you please! Leftover Greek Yogurt–Marinated Grilled Chicken (page 109) tastes great in this recipe.

BASIC NUTRITIONAL VALUES

Calories	310
Calories from Fat	120
Total Fat	13.0 g
Saturated Fat	2.7 g
Trans Fat	0.1 g
Cholesterol	85 mg
Sodium	490 mg
Potassium	510 mg
Total Carbohydrate	25 g
Dietary Fiber	4 g
Sugars	3 g
Protein	26 g
Phosphorus	305 mg

CHOICES/EXCHANGES

1 Starch, 1/2 Carbohydrate,
3 Lean Protein, 1 1/2 Fat

Mushroom Arugula Pizza

Mini pizzas are easy and fun to create using a sandwich thin and your favorite toppings.

INGREDIENTS

4 cloves garlic, chopped, divided
1/4 cup diced red onion
8 oz mushrooms, sliced
2 tsp olive oil
1 cup packed arugula (3 cups loose)
1/4 cup plus 1 Tbsp part-skim ricotta cheese
1/8 tsp white pepper
3 whole-wheat sandwich thins, split open
3 Tbsp reduced-fat shredded mozzarella

Prep Time: 15 minutes
Cook Time: 5 minutes
Serves: 6
Serving Size: 1 individual pizza (1/2 sandwich thin)

DIRECTIONS

1. In a skillet, sauté 2 cloves garlic, the onion, and mushrooms in olive oil for about 10 minutes or until mushrooms are golden brown.
2. In a food processor, combine arugula, ricotta, the remaining 2 cloves garlic, and white pepper and pulse until smooth.
3. Place 6 sandwich thin halves on baking pan.
4. Add 1 Tbsp of arugula mixture on each half of sandwich thin. Top with equal amounts of mushroom mixture and shredded mozzarella.
5. Broil for 5 minutes on low in the oven until cheese is melted.

BASIC NUTRITIONAL VALUES

Calories	100
Calories from Fat	35
Total Fat	**4.0 g**
Saturated Fat	1.2 g
Trans Fat	0.0 g
Cholesterol	**5 mg**
Sodium	**130 mg**
Potassium	**230 mg**
Total Carbohydrate	**14 g**
Dietary Fiber	3 g
Sugars	3 g
Protein	**6 g**
Phosphorus	**125 mg**

CHOICES/EXCHANGES

1 Starch, 1 Lean Protein

Sweet Potato Black Bean Chili

Slow cookers are great for all day cooking, and can also be useful for shorter durations when you need to step away from the kitchen for an hour or two.

INGREDIENTS

1 1/2 lb sweet potatoes
1 lb ground turkey breast
2 cups chopped onion
2 cloves garlic, crushed
1 Tbsp olive oil
2 (14.5-oz) cans diced tomatoes, undrained
1 (15.5-oz) can black beans, drained and rinsed
2 Tbsp chili powder
2 tsp cumin
1 tsp oregano
1 tsp hot pepper sauce (such as Tabasco; can use more for a spicier chili)

DIRECTIONS

1. Scrub sweet potatoes, poke hole in potatoes with a fork, and microwave for about 5 minutes until they begin to soften.
2. Cook turkey in a skillet for about 8 minutes. Once browned, add to slow cooker.
3. In the same skillet used for the turkey, sauté onion and garlic in olive oil for about 10 minutes until onion is softened. Add onion and garlic to slow cooker.
4. Cut softened sweet potatoes into small chunks and add to slow cooker.
5. Stir canned tomatoes, black beans, chili powder, cumin, oregano, and hot pepper sauce into slow cooker and cook for 2 hours.

Prep Time: 10 minutes
Cook Time: 2 hours
Serves: 8
Serving Size: 1 cup

BASIC NUTRITIONAL VALUES

Calories	**230**
Calories from Fat	25
Total Fat	**3.0 g**
Saturated Fat	0.5 g
Trans Fat	0.0 g
Cholesterol	**35 mg**
Sodium	**280 mg**
Potassium	**830 mg**
Total Carbohydrate	**34 g**
Dietary Fiber	8 g
Sugars	9 g
Protein	**19 g**
Phosphorus	**225 mg**

CHOICES/EXCHANGES

1 1/2 Starch, 2 Nonstarchy Vegetable, 2 Lean Protein

Tomato Red Pepper Soup with White Beans

We've put our own twist on classic tomato soup by giving it a boost with white beans, basil, and roasted red pepper.

Prep Time: 15 minutes
Cook Time: 25 minutes
Serves: 6
Serving Size: 1 cup

INGREDIENTS

2 tsp olive oil
1 cup finely diced onion
2 cloves garlic, minced
3 cups low-sodium vegetable broth
2 cups canned crushed tomatoes
1 (12-oz) jar roasted red peppers, drained, rinsed, and puréed in a food processor
1/4 cup chopped fresh basil
1 (14.5-oz) can reduced-sodium cannellini beans, drained and rinsed
6 tsp shredded Parmesan cheese, divided

DIRECTIONS

1. In a large soup pot, heat olive oil over medium heat. Add onions and sauté for 4–5 minutes until just starting to brown. Add garlic and cook for another 30 seconds.
2. Add broth and scrape any browned bits from bottom of the pan with your spoon. Add tomatoes and red peppers, and bring to a boil. Reduce heat, cover, and simmer for 15 minutes.
3. Add basil and beans, and simmer for an additional 5 minutes.
4. Serve hot with 1 tsp Parmesan cheese sprinkled on top of each serving.

BASIC NUTRITIONAL VALUES

Calories	**130**
Calories from Fat	20
Total Fat	**2.5 g**
Saturated Fat	0.4 g
Trans Fat	0.0 g
Cholesterol	**0 mg**
Sodium	**270 mg**
Potassium	**600 mg**
Total Carbohydrate	**23 g**
Dietary Fiber	6 g
Sugars	8 g
Protein	**6 g**
Phosphorus	**150 mg**

CHOICES/EXCHANGES

1 Starch, 2 Nonstarchy Vegetable

Hearty Turkey, Poblano, and Pumpkin Chili

We love chili during those "chilly" months of the year. This simple recipe provides a nice balance of veggies, lean protein, and fiber-packed beans.

Prep Time: 15 minutes
Cook Time: 15 minutes
Serves: 7
Serving Size: 1 cup chili, 2 Tbsp Greek yogurt, and 1 Tbsp cheese

INGREDIENTS

1 Tbsp canola oil
1/2 sweet onion, chopped
2 poblano peppers, chopped
1 lb 93% lean ground turkey
3 cloves garlic, chopped
1 1/2 Tbsp chili powder
2 Tbsp cumin
1 (14.5-oz) can kidney beans, drained and rinsed
1 (14.5-oz) can crushed tomatoes
1 (14.5-oz) can no-salt-added diced tomatoes
3/4 cup canned puréed pumpkin
1 Tbsp plus 1 tsp apple cider vinegar
14 Tbsp nonfat, plain Greek yogurt
7 Tbsp shredded sharp cheddar cheese

DIRECTIONS

1. In a large soup pot, heat canola oil over medium-high heat.
2. Add onion, poblano peppers, and turkey to pot. Cook for 5 minutes or until turkey is cooked through and vegetables have softened. Add garlic, chili powder, and cumin and cook for an additional 1–2 minutes.
3. Add beans and tomatoes. Cover pot, reduce heat to low, and simmer for 10 minutes.
4. Stir in pumpkin and vinegar and simmer for another 5 minutes.
5. Top each serving with 2 Tbsp Greek yogurt and 1 Tbsp cheddar cheese (or your other favorite chili fixings!).

BASIC NUTRITIONAL VALUES

Calories	280
Calories from Fat	90
Total Fat	10.0 g
Saturated Fat	3.1 g
Trans Fat	0.1 g
Cholesterol	60 mg
Sodium	290 mg
Potassium	830 mg
Total Carbohydrate	24 g
Dietary Fiber	6 g
Sugars	8 g
Protein	23 g
Phosphorus	315 mg

CHOICES/EXCHANGES

1 Starch, 2 Nonstarchy Vegetable, 2 Lean Protein, 1 1/2 Fat

Butternut Squash and Kale Soup

If you don't have an immersion blender to make this soup, you can use a regular blender to blend the vegetables and liquid together.

INGREDIENTS

1 large sweet onion, cut into wedges
4 cups cubed butternut squash (about 3/4-inch cubes)
1 Tbsp olive oil
Freshly ground black pepper, to taste
1 tsp dried thyme
1 (14.5-oz) can low-sodium chicken broth
3/4 cup water
3 cups chopped kale

Prep Time: 20 minutes
Cook Time: 35 minutes
Serves: 4
Serving Size: 1 cup

DIRECTIONS

1. Preheat oven to 425°F.
2. Line a large baking pan with aluminum foil and spread onion and squash over foil in a single layer. Drizzle vegetables with olive oil and toss lightly to coat; then season with pepper and thyme. Place in oven and bake for 30–35 minutes, or until vegetables are cooked through and starting to brown. Note: take vegetables out at least once in the middle of cooking to stir.
3. Combine roasted vegetables, chicken broth, and water in a large saucepan and use an immersion blender to blend ingredients together until smooth.
4. Heat blended soup over medium heat until heated through. Once heated through, stir in kale, and cook until wilted, about 3 minutes.

BASIC NUTRITIONAL VALUES

Calories	**130**
Calories from Fat	30
Total Fat	**3.5 g**
Saturated Fat	0.5 g
Trans Fat	0.0 g
Cholesterol	**0 mg**
Sodium	**75 mg**
Potassium	**740 mg**
Total Carbohydrate	**24 g**
Dietary Fiber	4 g
Sugars	8 g
Protein	**4 g**
Phosphorus	**110 mg**

CHOICES/EXCHANGES

1 Starch, 2 Nonstarchy Vegetable, 1/2 Fat

Chicken Tortilla Soup

Top this nutrient-packed soup with diced avocado or crumbled tortilla chips to pack an extra punch of flavor!

INGREDIENTS

Soup
2 tsp canola oil
1 medium onion, diced
1 poblano pepper, diced
1 medium zucchini, diced
2 cloves garlic, minced
1 Tbsp chili powder
1 tsp dried oregano
1 (4-oz) can green chiles, undrained
1 (28-oz) can crushed tomatoes
2 1/2 cups low-sodium chicken broth
1 (15-oz) can reduced-sodium black beans,
    drained and rinsed
1/2 cup frozen corn
2 cups shredded cooked chicken
1/2 cup fresh cilantro, chopped

Toppings
1 1/2 cups diced avocado
18 whole-grain tortilla chips

Prep Time: 25 minutes
Cook Time: 22 minutes
Serves: 6
Serving Size: 1 1/2 cups

DIRECTIONS

1. In a large soup pot, heat oil over medium-high heat. Add onion and poblano pepper and sauté for 2 minutes.

2. Add zucchini and sauté for another 5 minutes, or until vegetables have softened. Add garlic and sauté for another 30 seconds. Then, add all remaining soup ingredients except cilantro and stir to combine. Bring soup to a simmer, cover, and cook for 15 minutes.

3. Turn off heat, stir in cilantro, and cover again. Let soup sit for another 10 minutes before serving.

4. Top each serving with 1/4 cup diced avocado and 3 crumbled tortilla chips.

BASIC NUTRITIONAL VALUES	
Calories	**360**
Calories from Fat	130
Total Fat	**14.0 g**
Saturated Fat	2.4 g
Trans Fat	0.0 g
Cholesterol	**40 mg**
Sodium	**480 mg**
Potassium	**1190 mg**
Total Carbohydrate	**38 g**
Dietary Fiber	11 g
Sugars	11 g
Protein	**24 g**
Phosphorus	**300 mg**

CHOICES/EXCHANGES

1 Starch, 4 Nonstarchy Vegetable, 2 Lean Protein, 2 Fat

Chicken Salad Sliders

This lightened-up version of chicken salad uses tangy Greek yogurt and light mayonnaise along with other healthy, flavorful ingredients!

INGREDIENTS

2 cups chopped cooked chicken
1 celery stalk, finely diced
2 Tbsp finely diced red onion
1/3 cup dried cranberries
2 Tbsp unsalted, sliced almonds
1/4 cup nonfat, plain Greek yogurt
1/4 cup light mayonnaise
1 tsp Dijon mustard
Juice of 1/2 lemon
Freshly ground black pepper, to taste
6 whole-wheat slider buns
1 tomato, sliced into 6 slices

Prep Time: 20 minutes
Cook Time: N/A
Serves: 6
Serving Size: 1 whole-wheat bun, 1/3 cup chicken salad, and 1 tomato slice

DIRECTIONS

1. Mix all ingredients except buns and tomato slices in a medium mixing bowl.
2. Serve 1/3 cup chicken salad on each slider bun topped with 1 tomato slice.

Tip: You can also serve this chicken salad on lettuce wraps for fewer carbohydrates at mealtime!

BASIC NUTRITIONAL VALUES

Calories	**260**
Calories from Fat	80
Total Fat	**9.0 g**
Saturated Fat	1.6 g
Trans Fat	0.0 g
Cholesterol	**45 mg**
Sodium	**340 mg**
Potassium	**340 mg**
Total Carbohydrate	**28 g**
Dietary Fiber	4 g
Sugars	9 g
Protein	**18 g**
Phosphorus	**205 mg**

CHOICES/EXCHANGES

1 Starch, 1/2 Fruit, 1/2 Carbohydrate, 2 Lean Protein, 1/2 Fat

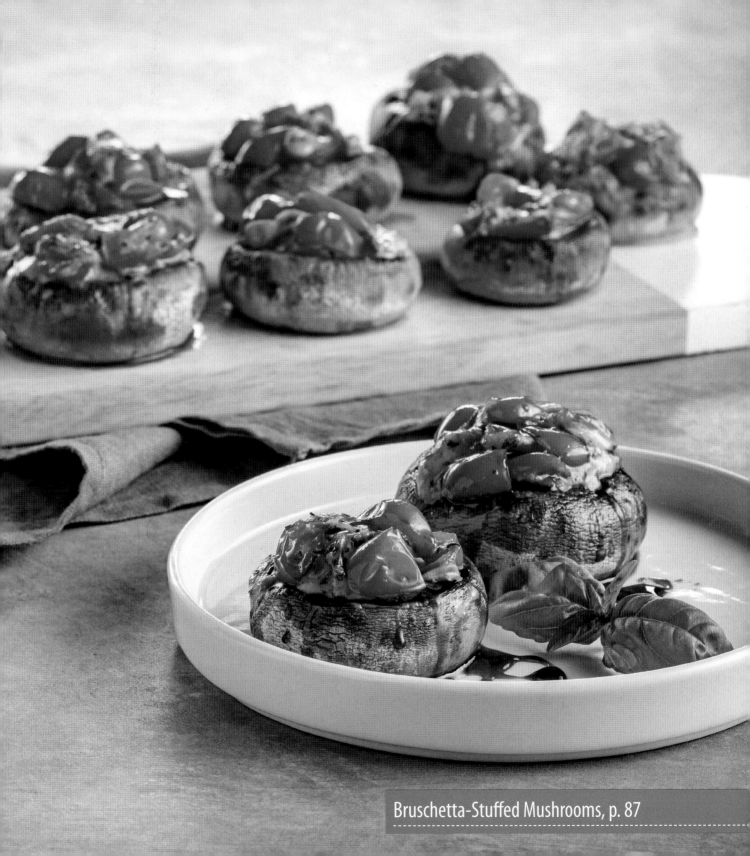

Bruschetta-Stuffed Mushrooms, p. 87

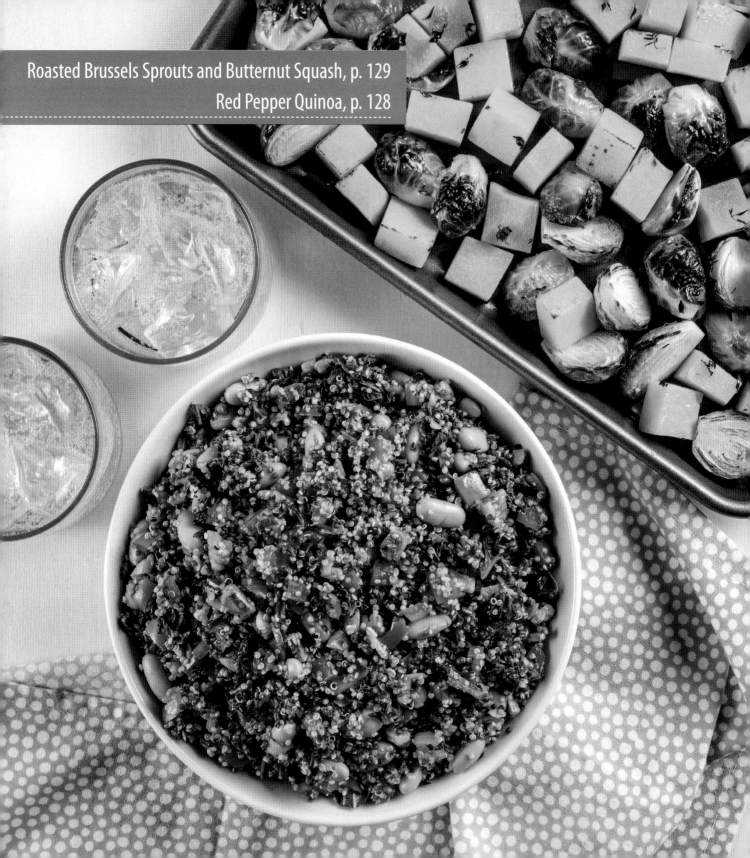

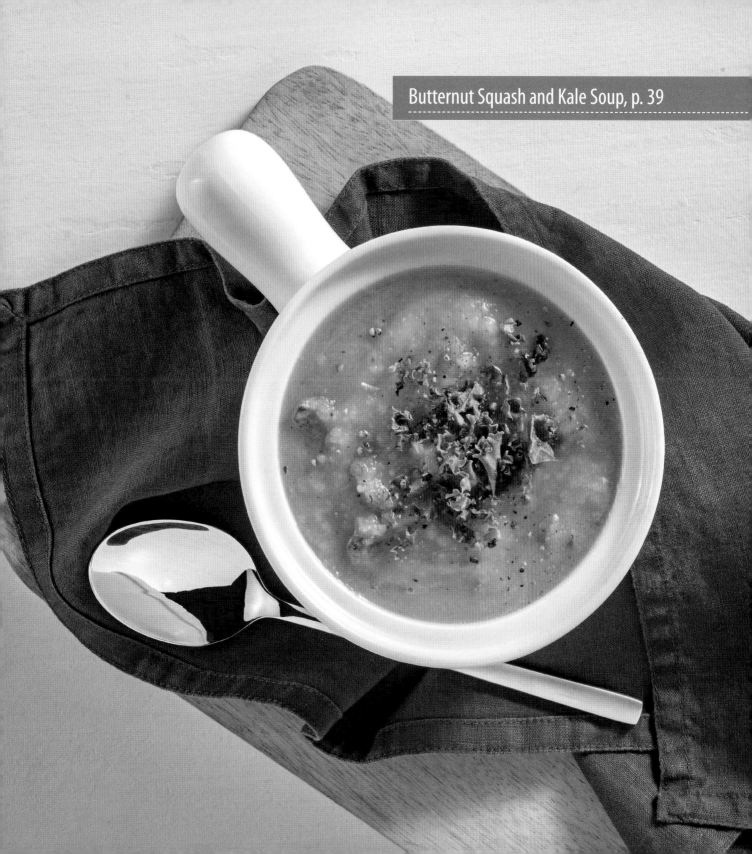

Butternut Squash and Kale Soup, p. 39

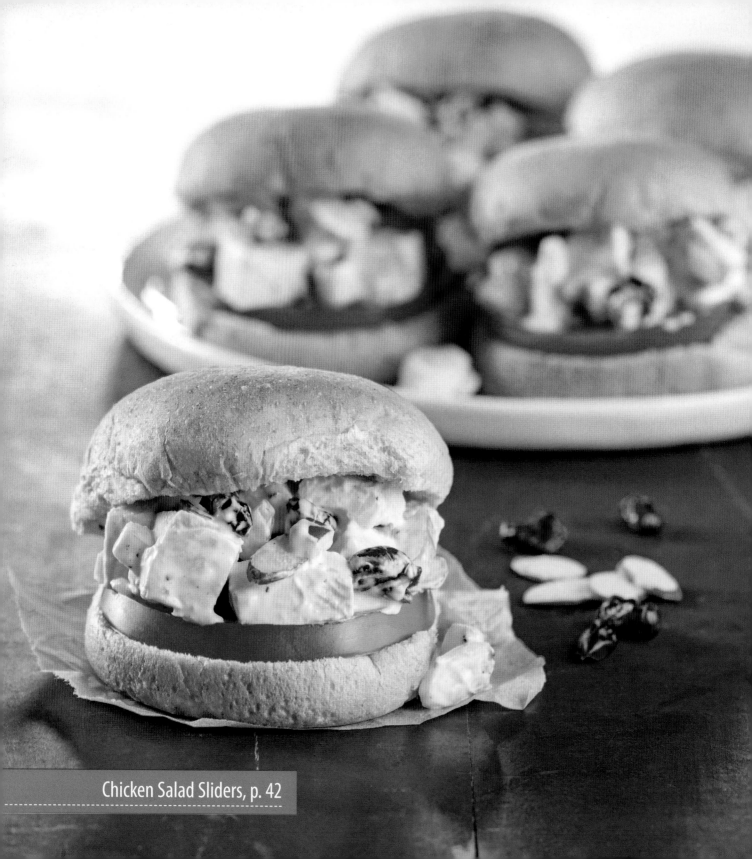
Chicken Salad Sliders, p. 42

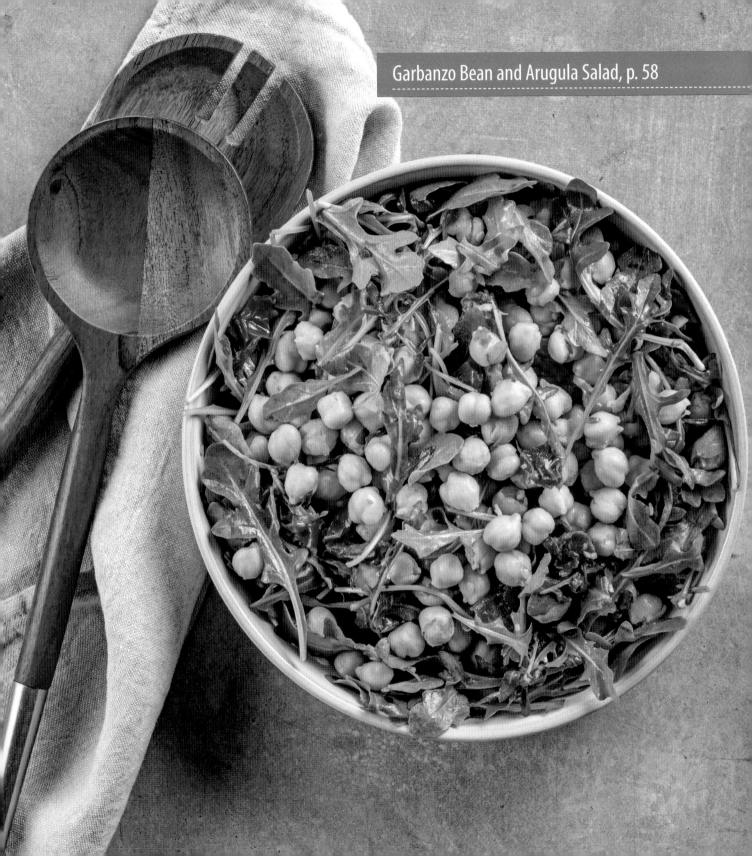

Garbanzo Bean and Arugula Salad, p. 58

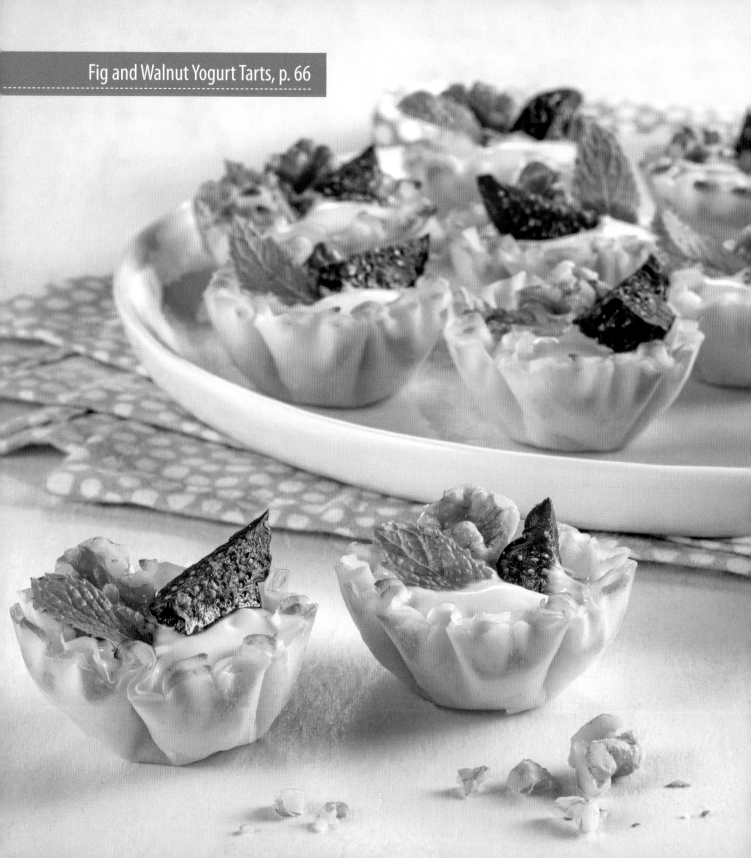

Fig and Walnut Yogurt Tarts, p. 66

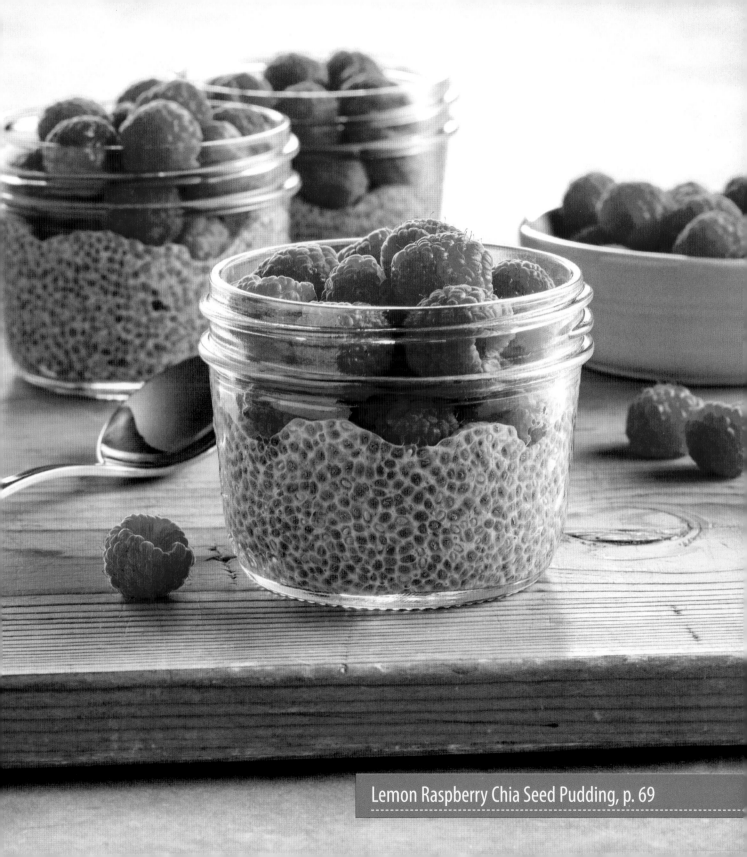

Lemon Raspberry Chia Seed Pudding, p. 69

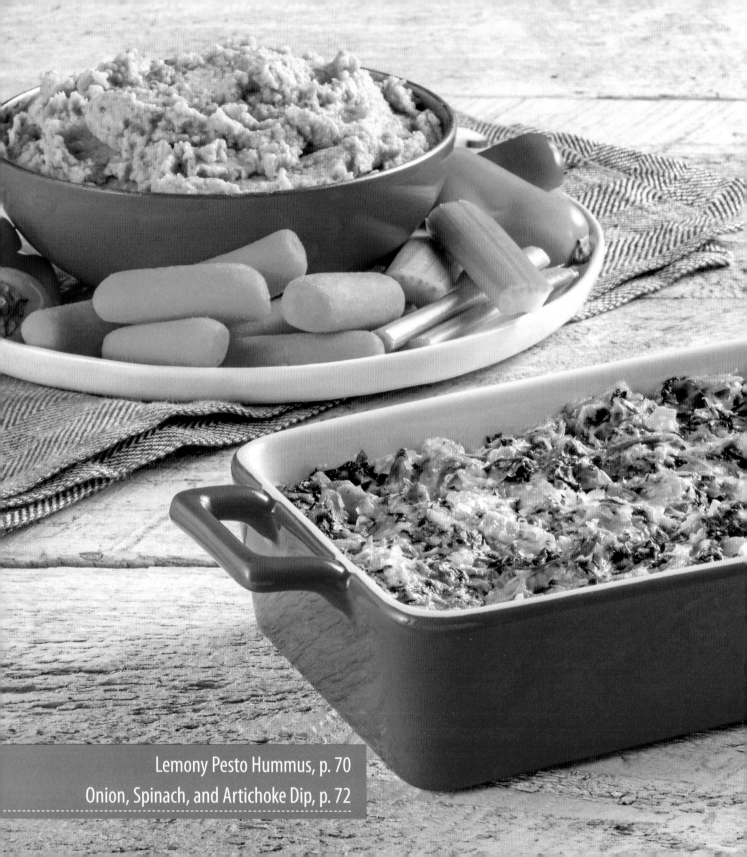

Lemony Pesto Hummus, p. 70
Onion, Spinach, and Artichoke Dip, p. 72

Creamy Chicken and Veggie Soup

This soup makes a delicious dinner during the chilly months of the year. To cut down on prep time, try buying some (or all) of the vegetables prechopped and using rotisserie chicken. If possible, opt for no-salt-added rotisserie chicken to keep sodium levels in check.

INGREDIENTS

2 tsp olive oil
1 tsp butter
1 cup chopped carrots
1 cup chopped onion
1 cup chopped celery
1/2 tsp dried thyme
Freshly ground black pepper, to taste
2 cloves garlic, minced
1/4 cup all-purpose flour
4 cups reduced-sodium chicken broth
2 bay leaves
2 cups broccoli florets
1 cup 2% milk
1 1/2 cups diced rotisserie or other precooked chicken breast

Prep Time: 10 minutes
Cook Time: 35 minutes
Serves: 7
Serving Size: 1 cup

DIRECTIONS

1. In a large soup pot, heat olive oil and butter over medium heat until butter is melted. Add carrots, onion, celery, thyme, and pepper and sauté for 5 minutes, stirring occasionally. Add garlic and cook for another minute. Vegetables should be starting to brown slightly.

2. Add flour and mix well to thoroughly coat vegetables. Cook about 1 minute and then whisk in broth, mixing well. Bring soup to a boil.

3. Add bay leaves and broccoli. Reduce heat, cover, and allow soup to simmer for 15 minutes.

4. Add milk and chicken and simmer for an additional 10 minutes with the top off, stirring occasionally until soup thickens slightly. Remove bay leaves and serve hot.

BASIC NUTRITIONAL VALUES

Calories	130
Calories from Fat	35
Total Fat	4.0 g
Saturated Fat	1.3 g
Trans Fat	0.1 g
Cholesterol	30 mg
Sodium	400 mg
Potassium	450 mg
Total Carbohydrate	11 g
Dietary Fiber	2 g
Sugars	5 g
Protein	14 g
Phosphorus	160 mg

CHOICES/EXCHANGES

1/2 Carbohydrate, 1 Nonstarchy Vegetable, 2 Lean Protein

Edamame Veggie Wrap

Pack this tasty wrap to go by wrapping it tightly in foil to hold the tortilla and veggie fillings together. Peel off the foil around the wrap as you eat for a mess-free lunch!

INGREDIENTS

1 Tbsp Tahini Sauce (page 25)
1 (6-inch) low-carb whole-wheat tortilla wrap
1/2 cup shelled edamame
1/4 cup halved grape tomatoes
3/4 cup mixed greens
Freshly ground black pepper, to taste

Prep Time: 5 minutes
Cook Time: N/A
Serves: 1
Serving Size: 1 wrap

DIRECTIONS

1. Spread Tahini Sauce over tortilla; then layer edamame, tomatoes, greens, and pepper over tahini.
2. Roll tortilla to make a wrap and enjoy!

BASIC NUTRITIONAL VALUES

Calories	**180**
Calories from Fat	70
Total Fat	**8.0 g**
Saturated Fat	0.9 g
Trans Fat	0.0 g
Cholesterol	**0 mg**
Sodium	**180 mg**
Potassium	**540 mg**
Total Carbohydrate	**21 g**
Dietary Fiber	12 g
Sugars	3 g
Protein	**14 g**
Phosphorus	**215 mg**

CHOICES/EXCHANGES

1 Starch, 1 Nonstarchy Vegetable,
1 Lean Protein, 1 Fat

Salads

Curried Tuna Salad

Give your everyday ho-hum tuna salad a unique twist by adding different spices and chopped vegetables.

INGREDIENTS

1 (5-oz) can tuna packed in water, drained
1/4 cup diced onion
1 stalk celery, diced
1/2 sweet red pepper, chopped
1/4 cup nonfat, plain Greek yogurt
2 Tbsp fresh lime juice (from 1 lime)
1 1/2 tsp yellow mustard
1/2 tsp freshly ground black pepper
1/2 tsp thyme
1/4 tsp curry powder
1/8 tsp garlic powder
Dash cayenne pepper, to taste
4 butter lettuce leaves
1 tomato, chopped
1/2 avocado, chopped

DIRECTIONS

1. In a large bowl, mix together all ingredients except lettuce, tomato, and avocado.
2. Place 1/4 cup of tuna mixture in each lettuce leaf.
3. Top each lettuce leaf with equal amounts of chopped tomato and avocado.

Prep Time: 15 minutes
Cook Time: N/A
Serves: 2
Serving Size: 1/2 cup salad, 2 lettuce leaves, 1/2 tomato, and 1/4 avocado

BASIC NUTRITIONAL VALUES

Calories	170
Calories from Fat	70
Total Fat	8.0 g
Saturated Fat	1.1 g
Trans Fat	0.0 g
Cholesterol	20 mg
Sodium	270 mg
Potassium	740 mg
Total Carbohydrate	14 g
Dietary Fiber	6 g
Sugars	6 g
Protein	16 g
Phosphorus	205 mg

CHOICES/EXCHANGES

1/2 Fruit, 2 Nonstarchy Vegetable, 2 Lean Protein

Farro, Tomato, and Basil Salad

This tasty salad has it all—juicy tomatoes, whole grains, punchy herbs, and protein-packed garbanzo beans, all lightly tossed with a balsamic vinaigrette and just the right amount of goat cheese. It's great on its own or served over greens for a light lunch!

INGREDIENTS

1/2 cup dry quick-cooking farro (to yield 1 cup cooked)
2 Tbsp olive oil
1 Tbsp balsamic vinegar
Juice of 1/2 lemon
Freshly ground black pepper, to taste
2 cups halved mini heirloom tomatoes or cherry tomatoes
1/3 cup chopped basil
1 cup drained and rinsed canned garbanzo beans (chickpeas)
1 oz goat cheese, crumbled

Prep Time: 10 minutes
Cook Time: 10 minutes
Serves: 8
Serving Size: 1/2 cup

DIRECTIONS

1. Cook farro according to package instructions.
2. While farro is cooking, whisk together olive oil, balsamic vinegar, lemon juice, and pepper in a small bowl. Set aside.
3. When farro is done, drain excess liquid and add to a large bowl. Then add tomatoes, basil, garbanzo beans, and balsamic vinaigrette. Toss salad ingredients together and top with crumbled goat cheese. Enjoy hot or cold.

BASIC NUTRITIONAL VALUES

Calories	**110**
Calories from Fat	45
Total Fat	**5.0 g**
Saturated Fat	1.1 g
Trans Fat	0.0 g
Cholesterol	**5 mg**
Sodium	**50 mg**
Potassium	**190 mg**
Total Carbohydrate	**14 g**
Dietary Fiber	3 g
Sugars	2 g
Protein	**4 g**
Phosphorus	**90 mg**

CHOICES/EXCHANGES

1 Starch, 1 Fat

Mixed Greens with Spicy Pecans, Goat Cheese, and Pear

This salad uses whole foods to create a mixture of sweet, savory, and spicy flavors.

INGREDIENTS

1 fresh medium pear (or apple)
2 dried figs
1 1/2 oz goat cheese, crumbled
8 cups mixed greens
1/2 cup chopped red onion
1/4 cup chopped Honey Spiced Pecans (page 68) or plain pecans
1/4 cup White Balsamic, Orange, and Chia Seed Dressing (page 26)

Prep Time: 10 minutes
Cook Time: N/A
Serves: 4
Serving Size: 2 cups salad and about 1 Tbsp dressing

DIRECTIONS

1. Slice pear and dried figs.
2. Divide goat cheese into 4 equal portions.
3. To assemble salad: Put 2 cups mixed greens in an individual serving bowl and top with 1/4 of the onion, 1/4 of the pear, 1/4 of the figs, 1 portion of goat cheese, and 1 Tbsp chopped pecans. Drizzle salad with 1 Tbsp dressing.
4. Repeat step 3 to make the remaining three salads.

BASIC NUTRITIONAL VALUES

Calories	**170**
Calories from Fat	100
Total Fat	**11.0 g**
Saturated Fat	2.5 g
Trans Fat	0.0 g
Cholesterol	**10 mg**
Sodium	**60 mg**
Potassium	**360 mg**
Total Carbohydrate	**17 g**
Dietary Fiber	5 g
Sugars	9 g
Protein	**4 g**
Phosphorus	**85 mg**

CHOICES/EXCHANGES

1/2 Fruit, 1 Nonstarchy Vegetable, 2 Fat

Mixed Greens with Strawberries, Feta, and Turkey Bacon

Bring this tasty salad to your next dinner party—it's simple and pairs well with many entrées!

INGREDIENTS

1 (5-oz) bag mixed greens
3 slices uncured cooked turkey bacon, chopped
1 1/4 cups sliced strawberries
1/4 cup feta cheese
1/4 cup White Balsamic Vinaigrette (page 27)
1/4 cup unsalted, sliced toasted almonds

Prep Time: 10 minutes
Cook Time: N/A
Serves: 6
Serving Size: 1 cup

DIRECTIONS

1. Combine greens, turkey bacon, strawberries, and feta cheese in a large salad bowl.
2. Toss with dressing and sprinkle with toasted almonds just before serving.

BASIC NUTRITIONAL VALUES

Calories	**100**
Calories from Fat	60
Total Fat	**7.0 g**
Saturated Fat	1.6 g
Trans Fat	0.1 g
Cholesterol	**10 mg**
Sodium	**120 mg**
Potassium	**170 mg**
Total Carbohydrate	**6 g**
Dietary Fiber	2 g
Sugars	4 g
Protein	**4 g**
Phosphorus	**70 mg**

CHOICES/EXCHANGES

1/2 Carbohydrate, 1 1/2 Fat

Quinoa, Arugula, and Apricot Salad

Pair this salad with our Simple Roasted Salmon (page 101) or Greek Yogurt–Marinated Grilled Chicken (page 109)!

INGREDIENTS

1 cup warm, cooked quinoa
8 whole dried apricots, chopped
1/4 cup diced onion
2 Tbsp toasted pine nuts
3 Tbsp feta cheese
Juice of 1/2 lemon
4 cups arugula
2 tsp olive oil, divided
Freshly ground black pepper, to taste

Prep Time: 10 minutes
Cook Time: N/A
Serves: 4
Serving Size: 1 cup arugula, 1/2 tsp olive oil, and 1/3 cup quinoa mixture

DIRECTIONS

1. In a small bowl, toss together quinoa, apricots, onion, pine nuts, feta cheese, and lemon juice.
2. Place 1 cup arugula in a salad bowl and drizzle with 1/2 tsp olive oil. Toss lightly to coat, then top with 1/4 of the quinoa mixture (about 1/3 cup) and season with pepper to taste.
3. Repeat for the remaining three salads.

Tip: One cup of dry quinoa results in 3 cups of cooked quinoa, so you can use any leftovers the next day to make our Black Bean Quinoa Cakes over Mixed Greens (page 56).

Up the flavor even more! Before step 1, sauté the onions in 1 tsp of olive oil with a clove of minced garlic. Then follow the recipe above.

BASIC NUTRITIONAL VALUES

Calories	170
Calories from Fat	70
Total Fat	**8.0 g**
Saturated Fat	1.7 g
Trans Fat	0.1 g
Cholesterol	**5 mg**
Sodium	**90 mg**
Potassium	**360 mg**
Total Carbohydrate	**21 g**
Dietary Fiber	3 g
Sugars	9 g
Protein	**5 g**
Phosphorus	**140 mg**

CHOICES/EXCHANGES

1 Starch, 1/2 Fruit, 1 1/2 Fat

Simple Salmon Salad

Use leftovers from our Simple Roasted Salmon recipe (page 101) to make this delicious, nutritious salad for lunch or dinner the following day.

INGREDIENTS

1 1/2 cups spinach
1/2 cup sliced cherry tomatoes
1/4 cup cooked quinoa
1 Tbsp feta cheese
3 oz Simple Roasted Salmon (page 101), warmed
1 Tbsp Homemade Balsamic Dressing (page 20)

Prep Time: 15 minutes
Cook Time: N/A
Serves: 1
Serving Size: 1 salad

DIRECTIONS

1. In a salad bowl, layer spinach, tomatoes, quinoa, and feta cheese. Top with warm salmon.
2. Drizzle with dressing and enjoy!

BASIC NUTRITIONAL VALUES

Calories	**360**
Calories from Fat	180
Total Fat	**20.0 g**
Saturated Fat	4.5 g
Trans Fat	0.1 g
Cholesterol	**70 mg**
Sodium	**230 mg**
Potassium	**970 mg**
Total Carbohydrate	**18 g**
Dietary Fiber	3 g
Sugars	6 g
Protein	**28 g**
Phosphorus	**440 mg**

CHOICES/EXCHANGES

1 Starch, 1 Nonstarchy Vegetable,
3 Lean Protein, 3 Fat

Spicy Peanut Broccoli Slaw

Using preshredded bags of slaw from the store saves lots of time on the preparation of any slaw.

INGREDIENTS

1 (10-oz) bag shredded broccoli slaw
1 bunch green onions, chopped (about 1/4 cup)
1/2 large red bell pepper, chopped (about 3/4 cup)
1/4 cup lightly salted cocktail peanuts, crushed (crush after measuring)
9 Tbsp Spicy Peanut Dressing (page 23)

Prep Time: 5 minutes
Cook Time: N/A
Serves: 6
Serving Size: 3/4 cup

DIRECTIONS

1. In a large bowl, mix broccoli slaw, onions, and red pepper together and set aside.
2. Sprinkle with crushed peanuts.
3. Serve slaw tossed in Spicy Peanut Dressing.

BASIC NUTRITIONAL VALUES

Calories	80
Calories from Fat	35
Total Fat	**4.0 g**
Saturated Fat	0.6 g
Trans Fat	0.0 g
Cholesterol	**0 mg**
Sodium	**110 mg**
Potassium	**300 mg**
Total Carbohydrate	**8 g**
Dietary Fiber	3 g
Sugars	3 g
Protein	**5 g**
Phosphorus	**85 mg**

CHOICES/EXCHANGES

1 Nonstarchy Vegetable, 1 Fat

Spinach, Avocado, and Summer Berry Salad

Pair this superfood-packed side dish with your favorite grilled chicken or fish recipe!

INGREDIENTS

10 oz fresh spinach
1 cup diced strawberries
1/2 cup blueberries
1 avocado, diced
1/3 cup finely diced red onion
6 Tbsp White Balsamic Vinaigrette (page 27)

Prep Time: 15 minutes
Cook Time: N/A
Serves: 8
Serving Size: 1 cup

DIRECTIONS

1. Place all ingredients through red onion in a large salad bowl.
2. Pour dressing over salad and toss to coat.

BASIC NUTRITIONAL VALUES

Calories	**90**
Calories from Fat	50
Total Fat	**6.0 g**
Saturated Fat	0.9 g
Trans Fat	0.0 g
Cholesterol	**0 mg**
Sodium	**30 mg**
Potassium	**350 mg**
Total Carbohydrate	**9 g**
Dietary Fiber	3 g
Sugars	4 g
Protein	**2 g**
Phosphorus	**35 mg**

CHOICES/EXCHANGES

1/2 Fruit, 1 Fat

Super Green Salad

This makes for a quick and tasty side dish that's sure to brighten up your meal! It's great for nights when you're entertaining or when you just need to get a veggie side dish on the table.

INGREDIENTS

4 cups baby spinach
1/4 cup sliced basil leaves
1 cup chopped cucumber
1 avocado, diced
1/4 cup shelled pistachios
1/4 cup Homemade Balsamic Dressing (page 20)

Prep Time: 10 minutes
Cook Time: N/A
Serves: 4
Serving Size: 1 salad

DIRECTIONS

1. In a large mixing bowl, toss together baby spinach, basil, cucumber, and avocado.
2. Place salad in 4 separate bowls and top each with 1 Tbsp pistachios and 1 Tbsp dressing.

BASIC NUTRITIONAL VALUES

Calories	**160**
Calories from Fat	130
Total Fat	**14.0 g**
Saturated Fat	1.9 g
Trans Fat	0.0 g
Cholesterol	**0 mg**
Sodium	**40 mg**
Potassium	**480 mg**
Total Carbohydrate	**9 g**
Dietary Fiber	4 g
Sugars	3 g
Protein	**3 g**
Phosphorus	**80 mg**

CHOICES/EXCHANGES

1/2 Carbohydrate, 3 Fat

Artichoke and Tomato Salad

Serve this as a side dish or serve on a bed of lettuce with garbanzo beans for a main dish.

INGREDIENTS

1 (14-oz) can whole artichoke hearts, drained and rinsed (do not use marinated artichokes)
1/2 cup thinly sliced red onion
1 cup chopped fresh tomato
2 Tbsp olive oil
3 Tbsp red wine vinegar

Prep Time: 5 minutes
Cook Time: N/A
Serves: 5
Serving Size: 1/2 cup

DIRECTIONS

1. Chop artichoke hearts in half.
2. Add artichokes, onion, and tomato to a salad bowl and mix gently.
3. In a small bowl, stir together olive oil and vinegar. Pour over artichoke mixture.

BASIC NUTRITIONAL VALUES

Calories	**90**
Calories from Fat	50
Total Fat	**6.0 g**
Saturated Fat	0.8 g
Trans Fat	0.0 g
Cholesterol	**0 mg**
Sodium	**140 mg**
Potassium	**230 mg**
Total Carbohydrate	**8 g**
Dietary Fiber	3 g
Sugars	2 g
Protein	**2 g**
Phosphorus	**45 mg**

CHOICES/EXCHANGES

2 Nonstarchy Vegetable, 1 Fat

Black Bean Quinoa Cakes over Mixed Greens

These Black Bean Quinoa Cakes make a tasty vegetarian meal!

INGREDIENTS

2 tsp olive oil
3/4 cup finely diced onion
2 cloves garlic, minced
1 (15-oz) can reduced-sodium black beans, drained and rinsed
1/2 cup water
1 Tbsp cumin
1/2 tsp smoked paprika
1 cup cooked quinoa
Nonstick cooking spray
2 (1-oz) slices sharp cheddar cheese, sliced into 4 equal squares
4 cups mixed greens
2 tomatoes, chopped
1/2 cup Avocado Cilantro Dressing (page 28)

Prep Time: 15 minutes
Cook Time: 30 minutes
Serves: 4
Serving Size: 2 black bean cakes, 1 cup of mixed greens, 1/2 chopped tomato, and 2 Tbsp dressing

DIRECTIONS

1. In a medium saucepan, heat olive oil over medium heat. Add onions and cook 3 minutes. Add garlic and cook 1 minute. Add beans, water, cumin, and paprika and bring to a simmer. Then cover the saucepan and cook an additional 8–10 minutes or until most of the liquid has been reduced and beans have softened.
2. Remove pan from heat and drain remaining liquid.

3. Use a potato masher to partially mash bean mixture, then stir in cooked quinoa.

4. Roll 1/4 cup of black bean–quinoa mixture into a ball and flatten to make a small cake or patty that is about 1/2 inch thick. Repeat with remaining black bean–quinoa mixture to make 8 patties.

5. Spray a large skillet with cooking spray and heat over medium-high heat. Cook patties 3–4 minutes on each side, topping each with a piece of cheese when you flip it.

6. To complete the meal, serve 2 black bean cakes over 1 cup mixed greens and 1/2 chopped tomato. Top salad with 2 Tbsp dressing.

BASIC NUTRITIONAL VALUES

Calories	**300**
Calories from Fat	120
Total Fat	**13.0 g**
Saturated Fat	4.2 g
Trans Fat	0.1 g
Cholesterol	**15 mg**
Sodium	**290 mg**
Potassium	**750 mg**
Total Carbohydrate	**35 g**
Dietary Fiber	10 g
Sugars	5 g
Protein	**13 g**
Phosphorus	**285 mg**

CHOICES/EXCHANGES

1 1/2 Starch, 2 Nonstarchy Vegetable, 1 Lean Protein, 2 Fat

Garbanzo Bean and Arugula Salad

This recipe is a simple and delicious combination of peppery arugula and sweet sundried tomatoes.

INGREDIENTS

1 (15.5-oz) can garbanzo beans (chickpeas), drained and rinsed
1/4 cup sundried tomatoes packed in olive oil and Italian herbs, drained
1 small clove garlic, crushed
2 cups fresh arugula (1/3 of 7-oz bag)

Prep Time: 15 minutes
Cook Time: N/A
Serves: 4
Serving Size: 3/4 cup

DIRECTIONS

1. Combine garbanzo beans, drained tomatoes, and garlic in a salad bowl.
2. Mix in arugula. Let sit for 10 minutes to slightly wilt arugula before serving.

BASIC NUTRITIONAL VALUES

Calories	**150**
Calories from Fat	40
Total Fat	**4.5 g**
Saturated Fat	0.4 g
Trans Fat	0.0 g
Cholesterol	**0 mg**
Sodium	**120 mg**
Potassium	**400 mg**
Total Carbohydrate	**22 g**
Dietary Fiber	6 g
Sugars	5 g
Protein	**7 g**
Phosphorus	**130 mg**

CHOICES/EXCHANGES

1 Starch, 1 Nonstarchy Vegetable,
1/2 Fat

Cucumber, Strawberry, and Feta Salad

This is a super-quick summer side that pairs perfectly with grilled chicken or fish!

INGREDIENTS

1 cucumber, diced (about 2 cups)
2/3 cup diced strawberries
1/4 cup chopped basil
1/4 cup feta cheese
Juice of 1/2 lime

Prep Time: 10 minutes
Cook Time: N/A
Serves: 4
Serving Size: 3/4 cup

DIRECTIONS

1. In a medium bowl, toss together cucumber, strawberries, basil, and feta cheese.
2. Top with lime juice, gently toss, and serve.

BASIC NUTRITIONAL VALUES

Calories	45
Calories from Fat	20
Total Fat	2.0 g
Saturated Fat	1.4 g
Trans Fat	0.1 g
Cholesterol	10 mg
Sodium	105 mg
Potassium	140 mg
Total Carbohydrate	5 g
Dietary Fiber	1 g
Sugars	3 g
Protein	2 g
Phosphorus	55 mg

CHOICES/EXCHANGES

1/2 Carbohydrate, 1/2 Fat

Snacks, Appetizers, and Desserts

Chocolate-Dipped Walnuts and Apricots

Satisfy your chocolate craving with dark chocolate–dipped nuts and dried fruit.

INGREDIENTS

1 oz dark chocolate
10 walnut halves
10 whole dried apricots

DIRECTIONS

1. Melt the dark chocolate in the microwave for 30 seconds, stir, and microwave for an additional 15–30 seconds until completely melted.
2. Dip one end of each walnut half and one end of each dried apricot into melted chocolate.
3. Lay dipped pieces on wax paper to harden. To speed up the hardening process, put the dipped fruit and nuts in the refrigerator.
4. Once chocolate has cooled and hardened, remove fruit and nuts from wax paper and enjoy.

Prep Time: 10 minutes
Cook Time: N/A
Serves: 5
Serving Size: 2 walnut halves and 2 apricots

BASIC NUTRITIONAL VALUES

Calories	**90**
Calories from Fat	40
Total Fat	**4.5 g**
Saturated Fat	1.3 g
Trans Fat	0.0 g
Cholesterol	**0 mg**
Sodium	**0 mg**
Potassium	**210 mg**
Total Carbohydrate	**12 g**
Dietary Fiber	2 g
Sugars	10 g
Protein	**1 g**
Phosphorus	**35 mg**

CHOICES/EXCHANGES

1/2 Fruit, 1/2 Carbohydrate, 1/2 Fat

Cinnamon Almond Butter Dip

We like this perfectly spiced dip with apple slices, but you can also enjoy it with pear slices or banana. Unlike many fruit dips, it's not overloaded with added sugar, and it even provides some protein for a more balanced snack!

INGREDIENTS

1/4 cup almond butter
1/2 cup nonfat, plain Greek yogurt
1/2 tsp cinnamon
1/4 tsp vanilla
1 tsp honey

Prep Time: 5 minutes
Cook Time: 30 seconds
Serves: 6
Serving Size: 2 Tbsp

DIRECTIONS

1. Place almond butter in a small microwave-safe bowl and heat for 20–30 seconds in the microwave or until melted. Transfer almond butter to a small food processor or blender and add Greek yogurt, cinnamon, and vanilla. Blend until smooth.
2. Transfer dip to a serving bowl and drizzle honey over top. Note: You can also mix the honey in if desired. Serve chilled.

BASIC NUTRITIONAL VALUES

Calories	**80**
Calories from Fat	50
Total Fat	**6.0 g**
Saturated Fat	0.5 g
Trans Fat	0.0 g
Cholesterol	**0 mg**
Sodium	**10 mg**
Potassium	**105 mg**
Total Carbohydrate	**4 g**
Dietary Fiber	1 g
Sugars	2 g
Protein	**4 g**
Phosphorus	**80 mg**

CHOICES/EXCHANGES

1 1/2 Fat

Cucumber Dill Dip

This is a light and fresh dip that's perfect for warmer weather. Serve it with raw veggies, whole-grain crackers, or pita chips.

INGREDIENTS

1/4 cup chopped cucumber
1/2 cup nonfat, plain Greek yogurt
1 tsp lemon juice
1/2 tsp dried dill

Prep Time: 10 minutes
Cook Time: N/A
Serves: 5
Serving Size: 2 Tbsp

DIRECTIONS

1. Add all ingredients to a food processor and process until mixed. Keep refrigerated until ready to serve.

BASIC NUTRITIONAL VALUES

Calories	15
Calories from Fat	0
Total Fat	**0.0 g**
Saturated Fat	0.0 g
Trans Fat	0.0 g
Cholesterol	**0 mg**
Sodium	**10 mg**
Potassium	**45 mg**
Total Carbohydrate	**1 g**
Dietary Fiber	0 g
Sugars	1 g
Protein	**2 g**
Phosphorus	**35 mg**

CHOICES/EXCHANGES

Free food

Fig and Walnut Yogurt Tarts

These beautiful yet simple tarts can be served as an appetizer or a snack.

INGREDIENTS

2 oz crumbled goat cheese
1/4 cup nonfat, plain Greek yogurt
2 Tbsp freshly squeezed clementine or orange juice
12 mini phyllo shells
4 mint leaves, each cut into 3 pieces
12 walnut halves
4 large figs (about 2 1/2 inches in diameter), each cut into 3 pieces

Prep Time: 15 minutes
Cook Time: N/A
Serves: 6
Serving Size: 2 tarts

DIRECTIONS

1. In a mixing bowl, mix goat cheese, yogurt, and orange juice together.
2. Fill each phyllo shell with 1 Tbsp of cheese mixture.
3. Top each with 1 piece of mint leaf, a walnut half, and a fig piece.
4. Keep refrigerated until ready to serve.

BASIC NUTRITIONAL VALUES

Calories	**130**
Calories from Fat	60
Total Fat	**7.0 g**
Saturated Fat	1.7 g
Trans Fat	0.0 g
Cholesterol	**10 mg**
Sodium	**60 mg**
Potassium	**150 mg**
Total Carbohydrate	**14 g**
Dietary Fiber	2 g
Sugars	8 g
Protein	**4 g**
Phosphorus	**65 mg**

CHOICES/EXCHANGES

1/2 Starch, 1/2 Fruit, 1 1/2 Fat

Fried Banana Yogurt

This dish is a quick and decadent-tasting afternoon snack or dessert.

INGREDIENTS

1 tsp canola or vegetable oil
1 banana (about 7 oz), sliced
1/4 tsp cinnamon
1 cup nonfat, plain Greek yogurt
2 Tbsp chopped pecans (1/2 oz)

Prep Time: 5 minutes
Cook Time: 5 minutes
Serves: 2
Serving Size: 1/2 cup yogurt, 1/2 banana, and 1 Tbsp pecans

DIRECTIONS

1. Heat oil in a nonstick pan over medium-low heat.
2. Slice banana and add to hot oil. Sprinkle with cinnamon. Cook for about 2 minutes until lightly browned on one side. Flip and cook for an additional 2 minutes.
3. Remove from heat and mix bananas into yogurt.
4. Top with chopped pecans.

BASIC NUTRITIONAL VALUES

Calories	**190**
Calories from Fat	70
Total Fat	**8.0 g**
Saturated Fat	0.8 g
Trans Fat	0.0 g
Cholesterol	**5 mg**
Sodium	**40 mg**
Potassium	**420 mg**
Total Carbohydrate	**20 g**
Dietary Fiber	2 g
Sugars	12 g
Protein	**13 g**
Phosphorus	**185 mg**

CHOICES/EXCHANGES

1 Fruit, 1/2 Fat-Free Milk,
1 Lean Protein, 1 Fat

Honey Spiced Pecans

These nuts are perfect for a quick snack or to add to a salad.

INGREDIENTS

1/4 tsp cumin
1/4 tsp cayenne pepper
1/4 tsp garlic powder
3/4 tsp ground cinnamon
3/4 tsp honey
1/2 tsp butter
2 tsp water
1 1/2 cups pecan halves

Prep Time: 10 minutes
Cook Time: 6 minutes
Serves: 12
Serving Size: 2 Tbsp

DIRECTIONS

1. Preheat oven to 300°F.
2. Mix cumin, cayenne pepper, garlic powder, and cinnamon together in a small bowl and set aside.
3. Place honey, butter, and water in microwave-safe dish and heat in microwave until melted, about 8 seconds.
4. Drizzle honey mixture over pecans, stirring to coat.
5. Place pecans on pan and bake for 3 minutes. Stir and bake for another 3 minutes. Watch carefully so pecans do not burn.
6. While hot from the oven, sprinkle spice blend over pecans and mix.

BASIC NUTRITIONAL VALUES

Calories	**90**
Calories from Fat	80
Total Fat	**9.0 g**
Saturated Fat	0.9 g
Trans Fat	0.0 g
Cholesterol	**0 mg**
Sodium	**0 mg**
Potassium	**55 mg**
Total Carbohydrate	**2 g**
Dietary Fiber	1 g
Sugars	1 g
Protein	**1 g**
Phosphorus	**35 mg**

CHOICES/EXCHANGES

2 Fat

Lemon Raspberry Chia Seed Pudding

This unique yet easy snack packs in heart-healthy omega-3 fatty acids from the chia seeds along with other nutrition bonuses like protein and fiber.

INGREDIENTS

1/4 cup chia seeds
1 cup unsweetened vanilla almond milk
1/2 tsp lemon zest
1 1/2 tsp lemon juice
1 Tbsp honey
2 cups raspberries

Prep Time: 5 minutes
Refrigeration Time: 1 hour
Cook Time: N/A
Serves: 4
Serving Size: 1/3 cup pudding and 1/2 cup raspberries

DIRECTIONS

1. In a small mixing bowl or large mason jar, whisk together all ingredients except raspberries. Put mixture in the refrigerator for at least an hour until chia seeds soak up liquid and it becomes a pudding consistency.
2. To serve, put 1/3 cup chia seed pudding in a small bowl and top with 1/2 cup raspberries.

BASIC NUTRITIONAL VALUES

Calories	120
Calories from Fat	45
Total Fat	**5.0 g**
Saturated Fat	0.5 g
Trans Fat	0.0 g
Cholesterol	**0 mg**
Sodium	**50 mg**
Potassium	**200 mg**
Total Carbohydrate	**18 g**
Dietary Fiber	9 g
Sugars	7 g
Protein	**3 g**
Phosphorus	**135 mg**

CHOICES/EXCHANGES

1/2 Fruit, 1/2 Carbohydrate, 1 Fat

Lemony Pesto Hummus

Enjoy this hummus as a dip for snacking with nonstarchy vegetables, whole-wheat pita, or whole-grain crackers.

INGREDIENTS

1 (14.5-oz) can garbanzo beans (chickpeas), drained and rinsed
2 Tbsp store-bought pesto
Juice of 1 small lemon (or 1/2 large lemon)
1/2 tsp freshly ground black pepper

Prep Time: 5 minutes
Cook Time: N/A
Serves: 5
Serving Size: 1/4 cup

DIRECTIONS

1. Add all ingredients to a food processor or blender. Blend until thoroughly mixed.

BASIC NUTRITIONAL VALUES

Calories	**100**
Calories from Fat	25
Total Fat	**3.0 g**
Saturated Fat	0.4 g
Trans Fat	0.0 g
Cholesterol	**0 mg**
Sodium	**150 mg**
Potassium	**150 mg**
Total Carbohydrate	**14 g**
Dietary Fiber	4 g
Sugars	3 g
Protein	**5 g**
Phosphorus	**80 mg**

CHOICES/EXCHANGES

1 Starch, 1/2 Fat

Mango Freeze

This makes for a delicious, frozen whole-food treat on a hot summer afternoon.

INGREDIENTS

1 cup frozen mango chunks
1/2 tsp minced fresh ginger
2 Tbsp unsweetened vanilla almond milk
2 Tbsp nonfat, vanilla Greek yogurt
1/4 tsp vanilla
1 tsp unsweetened coconut, toasted
8 pistachios, chopped

Prep Time: 5 minutes
Cook Time: N/A
Serves: 2
Serving Size: 1/2 cup mango freeze, 4 pistachios, and 1/2 tsp coconut

DIRECTIONS

1. Blend mango, ginger, almond milk, yogurt, and vanilla in a food processor or blender until smooth. Note: You can let mango sit out a few minutes first, but it should still be frozen for blending.
2. Divide mango mixture between two bowls, and top with coconut and pistachios. Serve immediately.

BASIC NUTRITIONAL VALUES

Calories	90
Calories from Fat	20
Total Fat	**2.5 g**
Saturated Fat	0.7 g
Trans Fat	0.0 g
Cholesterol	**0 mg**
Sodium	**20 mg**
Potassium	**220 mg**
Total Carbohydrate	**18 g**
Dietary Fiber	2 g
Sugars	15 g
Protein	**2 g**
Phosphorus	**45 mg**

CHOICES/EXCHANGES

1 Fruit, 1/2 Fat

Onion, Spinach, and Artichoke Dip

Enjoy this dip with fresh-cut vegetables such as baby carrots, celery sticks, sliced cucumbers, or mini bell peppers. It's a simple way to incorporate more vegetables (and therefore, more nutrients) into your next party spread!

INGREDIENTS

1 tsp olive oil
1 onion, finely diced
1 (15-oz) can artichoke hearts, drained and rinsed
1/2 tsp dried thyme
1 (6-oz) bag fresh spinach, coarsely chopped
1/4 cup light mayonnaise
4 light spreadable cheese wedges (such as Laughing Cow)
2 Tbsp freshly grated Parmesan cheese, divided
Juice of 1 lemon

Prep Time: 15 minutes
Cook Time: 15 minutes
Serves: 20
Serving Size: 2 Tbsp

DIRECTIONS

1. Preheat oven to 350°F.
2. In a large skillet, heat olive oil over medium heat. Add onion and sauté for 5 minutes, stirring frequently. Add artichokes and thyme and cook for an additional 3 minutes or until veggies begin to brown. Add spinach and cook for an additional 1–2 minutes or until spinach is wilted. Remove skillet from heat.

3. In a small microwave-safe bowl, combine light mayonnaise, cheese wedges, and 1 Tbsp Parmesan cheese. Heat in microwave for 30 seconds to soften and then mix well. Note: If needed, heat mixture in 15-second increments until cheeses are softened and easily mixed with mayonnaise.

4. Add cheese mixture and lemon juice to sautéed vegetables and mix well.

5. Spread dip into a small baking dish, top with remaining 1 Tbsp of Parmesan cheese, and bake in the oven for 5 minutes.

BASIC NUTRITIONAL VALUES

Calories	35
Calories from Fat	20
Total Fat	**2.0 g**
Saturated Fat	0.7 g
Trans Fat	0.0 g
Cholesterol	**2 mg**
Sodium	**115 mg**
Potassium	**110 mg**
Total Carbohydrate	**3 g**
Dietary Fiber	1 g
Sugars	1 g
Protein	**1 g**
Phosphorus	**40 mg**

CHOICES/EXCHANGES

1/2 Fat

Peanut Butter and Oatmeal Energy Bites

These perfectly pre-portioned snacks are great when you're on your way out the door but need a quick pick-me-up. We like them just before a walk or workout!

INGREDIENTS

1/3 cup smooth natural peanut butter
2 Tbsp honey
3/4 tsp vanilla
1 tsp canola oil
1 cup quick oats
1/4 cup dried cranberries

Prep Time: 10 minutes
Cook Time: N/A
Serves: 6
Serving Size: 3 bites

DIRECTIONS

1. In a small microwave-safe ramekin, heat peanut butter in the microwave for 20–30 seconds or until melted.
2. In a small mixing bowl, combine melted peanut butter, honey, vanilla, and canola oil and mix until thoroughly combined.
3. Add oats and dried cranberries and stir until dry ingredients are evenly coated with peanut butter mixture.
4. Scoop batter into 1 Tbsp portions and roll into balls. Store in the refrigerator in a tightly sealed container.

BASIC NUTRITIONAL VALUES

Calories	**180**
Calories from Fat	80
Total Fat	**9.0 g**
Saturated Fat	1.1 g
Trans Fat	0.0 g
Cholesterol	**0 mg**
Sodium	**55 mg**
Potassium	**150 mg**
Total Carbohydrate	**22 g**
Dietary Fiber	3 g
Sugars	10 g
Protein	**5 g**
Phosphorus	**110 mg**

CHOICES/EXCHANGES

1/2 Starch, 1 Carbohydrate,
1 1/2 Fat

Pumpkin Hummus

Pair this tasty hummus with fresh veggies or pita chips—or enjoy it on toast for a quick snack!

INGREDIENTS

1 (15-oz) can garbanzo beans (chickpeas), drained and rinsed
1/2 cup canned pumpkin
2 Tbsp tahini
1 Tbsp olive oil
1 Tbsp lemon juice
2 cloves garlic
1/4 tsp smoked paprika
Freshly ground black pepper, to taste

Prep Time: 10 minutes
Cook Time: N/A
Serves: 7
Serving Size: 1/4 cup

DIRECTIONS

1. Add all ingredients to a food processor or blender and blend until smooth.

BASIC NUTRITIONAL VALUES

Calories	**110**
Calories from Fat	45
Total Fat	**5.0 g**
Saturated Fat	0.7 g
Trans Fat	0.0 g
Cholesterol	**0 mg**
Sodium	**70 mg**
Potassium	**160 mg**
Total Carbohydrate	**13 g**
Dietary Fiber	4 g
Sugars	3 g
Protein	**4 g**
Phosphorus	**100 mg**

CHOICES/EXCHANGES

1 Starch, 1 Fat

Quick Cinnamon Baked Apple

There is nothing easier than turning an ordinary piece of fruit into a delicious dessert. Try serving this recipe with the Yogurt Topping (page 82)!

INGREDIENTS

1 medium apple (McIntosh or other cooking apple)
2 tsp whipped butter
1 tsp brown sugar
1/2 tsp ground cinnamon

Prep Time: 5 minutes
Cook Time: 20 minutes
Serves: 2
Serving Size: 1/2 apple

DIRECTIONS

1. Preheat oven to 375°F.
2. Peel and core the apple and cut it in half.
3. Put 1 tsp whipped butter in the center of each apple half.
4. Sprinkle each apple half with 1/2 tsp brown sugar and 1/4 tsp cinnamon.
5. Bake in the oven for 15–20 minutes, or until apple is soft.
6. Serve warm and top with Yogurt Topping (page 82), if desired.

BASIC NUTRITIONAL VALUES

Calories	60
Calories from Fat	20
Total Fat	**2.0 g**
Saturated Fat	1.2 g
Trans Fat	0.0 g
Cholesterol	**5 mg**
Sodium	**15 mg**
Potassium	**65 mg**
Total Carbohydrate	**11 g**
Dietary Fiber	1 g
Sugars	9 g
Protein	**0 g**
Phosphorus	**10 mg**

CHOICES/EXCHANGES

1/2 Fruit, 1/2 Fat

Raspberry Mint–Infused Water

Flavored water is a refreshing and delicious alternative to diet soda. Try different combinations of herbs and fruit to create your own favorites.

INGREDIENTS

10 fresh mint leaves
4 cups water
1/2 cup fresh raspberries

Prep Time: 5 minutes
Cook Time: N/A
Serves: 4
Serving Size: 1 cup

DIRECTIONS

1. Chop mint leaves and add to a pitcher with the water. Add whole raspberries to the pitcher as well.
2. Allow water to sit in the refrigerator to let the flavors infuse. The longer it sits, the more flavorful it will be. Enjoy cold.

BASIC NUTRITIONAL VALUES

Calories	**10**
Calories from Fat	0
Total Fat	**0.0 g**
Saturated Fat	0.0 g
Trans Fat	0.0 g
Cholesterol	**0 mg**
Sodium	**10 mg**
Potassium	**25 mg**
Total Carbohydrate	**2 g**
Dietary Fiber	1 g
Sugars	1 g
Protein	**0 g**
Phosphorus	**5 mg**

CHOICES/EXCHANGES

Free food

Roasted Red Pepper Spread

Add variety to your superfood snack selection with this tasty all-purpose spread. It's great on whole-grain crackers or with fresh veggies like carrots, celery, cucumber, or mini bell peppers. You can also enjoy it as a spread on sandwiches or wraps!

INGREDIENTS

1 Tbsp olive oil
1 clove garlic
1 cup cubed day-old bread (large, unseasoned croutons will also work)
1 roasted red pepper, drained, rinsed, and patted dry with a paper towel
1 Tbsp chopped parsley
2 Tbsp chopped walnuts
1/4 cup nonfat, plain Greek yogurt

Prep Time: 5 minutes
Cook Time: N/A
Serves: 6
Serving Size: 2 Tbsp

DIRECTIONS

1. In a small food processor, combine all ingredients except Greek yogurt. Blend until thoroughly chopped and mixed.
2. Add Greek yogurt to food processor and blend until smooth.

BASIC NUTRITIONAL VALUES

Calories	**60**
Calories from Fat	35
Total Fat	**4.0 g**
Saturated Fat	0.5 g
Trans Fat	0.0 g
Cholesterol	**0 mg**
Sodium	**55 mg**
Potassium	**50 mg**
Total Carbohydrate	**5 g**
Dietary Fiber	0 g
Sugars	1 g
Protein	**2 g**
Phosphorus	**30 mg**

CHOICES/EXCHANGES

1/2 Carbohydrate, 1/2 Fat

Spiced Cranberry Hot Tea

Enjoy the naturally sweet and tart flavor and the wonderful aroma of this tea. It's a low-calorie and flavorful alternative to sugar-laden tea or coffee drinks.

INGREDIENTS

4 cups water
2 cinnamon sticks
1 Tbsp sliced fresh ginger
1/4 cup fresh cranberries

Prep Time: 5 minutes
Cook Time: 15 minutes
Serves: 4
Serving Size: 1 cup

DIRECTIONS

1. Place all ingredients in saucepan and simmer, covered, on low heat until cranberries burst and liquid is pink. To infuse a stronger flavor, let the tea sit after cranberries burst.
2. Remove from heat and strain.

BASIC NUTRITIONAL VALUES

Calories	**0**
Calories from Fat	0
Total Fat	**0.0 g**
Saturated Fat	0.0 g
Trans Fat	0.0 g
Cholesterol	**0 mg**
Sodium	**10 mg**
Potassium	**0 mg**
Total Carbohydrate	**0 g**
Dietary Fiber	0 g
Sugars	0 g
Protein	**0 g**
Phosphorus	**0 mg**

CHOICES/EXCHANGES

Free food

Orange Ginger Hot Tea

This is a light, spicy fruit tea that can be served hot or cold.

INGREDIENTS

4 cups water
3 orange slices
1 (1-inch) piece fresh ginger, peeled and sliced
5 whole cloves

Prep Time: 5 minutes
Cook Time: 15 minutes
Serves: 4
Serving Size: 1 cup

DIRECTIONS

1. Bring water to a boil in a saucepan.
2. Add orange, ginger, and cloves and reduce heat to low. Cover and let simmer for about 15 minutes. To infuse a stronger flavor, let the tea sit after simmering.
3. Remove from heat and strain.

BASIC NUTRITIONAL VALUES

Calories	5
Calories from Fat	0
Total Fat	**0.0 g**
Saturated Fat	0.0 g
Trans Fat	0.0 g
Cholesterol	**0 mg**
Sodium	**10 mg**
Potassium	**15 mg**
Total Carbohydrate	**1 g**
Dietary Fiber	0 g
Sugars	1 g
Protein	**0 g**
Phosphorus	**0 mg**

CHOICES/EXCHANGES

Free food

Sunflower Granola

This is a quick-to-prepare, slightly sweet granola that is great by itself, with almond milk, or mixed with yogurt and fresh fruit.

INGREDIENTS

1/2 cup rolled oats
1/4 cup raw sunflower seeds
1/4 cup raisins
1/2 tsp cinnamon
2 tsp honey
1 tsp canola oil
1 Tbsp whole flaxseeds

Prep Time: 10 minutes
Cook Time: 15 minutes
Serves: 8
Serving Size: 2 Tbsp

DIRECTIONS

1. Preheat oven to 300°F.
2. In a large bowl, mix all ingredients together.
3. Spread granola mixture on a pan or baking sheet.
4. Bake for 15 minutes total, stirring every 5 minutes.

BASIC NUTRITIONAL VALUES

Calories	**80**
Calories from Fat	30
Total Fat	**3.5 g**
Saturated Fat	0.4 g
Trans Fat	0.0 g
Cholesterol	**0 mg**
Sodium	**0 mg**
Potassium	**95 mg**
Total Carbohydrate	**10 g**
Dietary Fiber	2 g
Sugars	4 g
Protein	**2 g**
Phosphorus	**65 mg**

CHOICES/EXCHANGES

1/2 Carbohydrate, 1 Fat

Yogurt Topping

Add a quick, crunchy topping to grilled fruit or try it on Quick Cinnamon Baked Apples (page 76).

INGREDIENTS

2 Tbsp Sunflower Granola (page 81)
1/4 cup nonfat, plain Greek yogurt

DIRECTIONS

1. In a small bowl, mix granola and yogurt together.

Prep Time: 5 minutes
Cook Time: N/A
Serves: 1
Serving Size: 6 Tbsp

BASIC NUTRITIONAL VALUES

Calories	**110**
Calories from Fat	35
Total Fat	**4.0 g**
Saturated Fat	0.4 g
Trans Fat	0.0 g
Cholesterol	**4 mg**
Sodium	**20 mg**
Potassium	**180 mg**
Total Carbohydrate	**12 g**
Dietary Fiber	2 g
Sugars	6 g
Protein	**8 g**
Phosphorus	**140 mg**

CHOICES/EXCHANGES

1/2 Fat-Free Milk,
1/2 Carbohydrate, 1 Fat

Sweet Potato Fries

Make your own healthier fries that both adults and kids will love!

INGREDIENTS

1 1/2 lb sweet potatoes
1 Tbsp olive oil
Freshly ground black pepper, to taste

DIRECTIONS

1. Preheat oven to 350°F.
2. Scrub sweet potatoes and cut into about 30 equal-sized pieces.
3. Coat potato pieces with olive oil.
4. Place on baking sheet and bake for 20 minutes. Turn fries halfway through baking to brown on both slides. Potatoes are done when soft.
5. Sprinkle fries with pepper. Serve with Rosemary Honey Mustard Dipping Sauce (page 22), if desired.

Prep Time: 10 minutes
Cook Time: 20 minutes
Serves: 5
Serving Size: 6 fries

BASIC NUTRITIONAL VALUES

Calories	**120**
Calories from Fat	25
Total Fat	**3.0 g**
Saturated Fat	0.4 g
Trans Fat	0.0 g
Cholesterol	**0 mg**
Sodium	**40 mg**
Potassium	**520 mg**
Total Carbohydrate	**23 g**
Dietary Fiber	4 g
Sugars	7 g
Protein	**2 g**
Phosphorus	**60 mg**

CHOICES/EXCHANGES

1 1/2 Starch

4-Ingredient Guacamole

Have this guacamole as a snack with whole-wheat crackers, baby carrots, or cucumber rounds. You can also use it as a condiment for your tacos, burgers, or sandwiches.

INGREDIENTS

1 medium avocado
Juice of 1/2 lime
2 Tbsp canned chopped green chiles
2 Tbsp finely diced red onion

Prep Time: 5 minutes
Cook Time: N/A
Serves: 4
Serving Size: 1/4 cup

DIRECTIONS

1. Peel avocado and remove the pit.
2. In a medium bowl, partially mash avocado so that some small chunks remain.
3. Stir in lime juice, green chiles, and red onion.

BASIC NUTRITIONAL VALUES

Calories	**70**
Calories from Fat	50
Total Fat	**6.0 g**
Saturated Fat	0.8 g
Trans Fat	0.0 g
Cholesterol	**0 mg**
Sodium	**25 mg**
Potassium	**210 mg**
Total Carbohydrate	**4 g**
Dietary Fiber	3 g
Sugars	1 g
Protein	**1 g**
Phosphorus	**25 mg**

CHOICES/EXCHANGES

1 1/2 Fat

Slow-Cooker Almond Rice Pudding

Enjoy this delicious rice pudding made from whole-grain rice and sweetened with fruit and spices.

INGREDIENTS

1/3 cup dry brown rice
3 cups unsweetened vanilla almond milk
6 dates, chopped in small pieces
1 cup canned pineapple, drained
2 cinnamon sticks
1 tsp vanilla extract
6 Tbsp unsalted, sliced almonds
1/4 tsp cinnamon

Prep Time: 10 minutes
Cook Time: 4 hours (on high) in slow cooker plus 6 minutes
Serves: 6
Serving Size: 1/2 cup pudding, 1 Tbsp almonds, and a dash of cinnamon

DIRECTIONS

1. In slow cooker, combine rice, almond milk, dates, pineapple, and cinnamon sticks.
2. Stir and cook on high for 4 hours.
3. Remove from heat, remove cinnamon sticks (and discard), and stir in vanilla.
4. Place almonds on a baking sheet. Toast almonds by baking at 350°F for about 6 minutes, shaking baking sheet every 2 minutes to prevent burning.
5. Sprinkle the top of the pudding with cinnamon and almonds.

BASIC NUTRITIONAL VALUES

Calories	**130**
Calories from Fat	45
Total Fat	**5.0 g**
Saturated Fat	0.5 g
Trans Fat	0.0 g
Cholesterol	**0 mg**
Sodium	**90 mg**
Potassium	**250 mg**
Total Carbohydrate	**20 g**
Dietary Fiber	3 g
Sugars	9 g
Protein	**3 g**
Phosphorus	**75 mg**

CHOICES/EXCHANGES

1/2 Starch, 1 Fruit, 1 Fat

Banana Cinnamon "Fro-Yo"

This quick, homemade "frozen yogurt" provides fiber, potassium, and some calcium from the almond milk and Greek yogurt! Keep leftovers in the freezer in an airtight container for 3–4 days after you make it and enjoy for an afternoon snack or sweet after dinner.

INGREDIENTS

2 medium frozen bananas
1/3 cup unsweetened vanilla almond milk
1/3 cup nonfat, plain Greek yogurt
1/2 tsp ground cinnamon

Prep Time: 5 minutes
Cook Time: N/A
Serves: 3
Serving Size: 1/2 cup

DIRECTIONS

1. In a small food processor or blender, combine all ingredients. Blend until ingredients are thoroughly combined and frozen yogurt is the consistency of soft-serve ice cream.
2. Serve immediately or transfer to a container with an airtight lid and store in the freezer.

BASIC NUTRITIONAL VALUES

Calories	**100**
Calories from Fat	10
Total Fat	**1.0 g**
Saturated Fat	0.2 g
Trans Fat	0.0 g
Cholesterol	**0 mg**
Sodium	**30 mg**
Potassium	**370 mg**
Total Carbohydrate	**21 g**
Dietary Fiber	3 g
Sugars	11 g
Protein	**4 g**
Phosphorus	**55 mg**

CHOICES/EXCHANGES

1 1/2 Fruit

Bruschetta-Stuffed Mushrooms

Bruschetta is a colorful and delicious appetizer for any gathering. For a lower-carb option, try this simple bruschetta stuffed in mushrooms instead of serving it on the traditional baguette.

INGREDIENTS

1 pint grape tomatoes
2 tsp olive oil
2 cloves garlic, chopped
2 tsp dried basil
1/3 cup 2% mozzarella cheese
2 Tbsp freshly grated Parmesan cheese
1 (14-oz) pack stuffer (larger) mushrooms
1 Tbsp balsamic vinegar

Prep Time: 10 minutes
Cook Time: 20 minutes
Serves: 7
Serving Size: 2 mushroom caps

DIRECTIONS

1. Cut tomatoes into quarters. Set aside.
2. In a skillet, heat olive oil and add garlic. Sauté garlic for about 1 minute.
3. Add tomatoes and continue to sauté for about 4 minutes.
4. Remove from heat and stir in basil and both cheeses.
5. Remove stems from mushrooms and fill with tomato mixture.
6. Bake in oven for 15 minutes at 350°F.
7. Let cool slightly and drizzle with balsamic vinegar. Serve warm.

BASIC NUTRITIONAL VALUES

Calories	**50**
Calories from Fat	25
Total Fat	**3.0 g**
Saturated Fat	1.0 g
Trans Fat	0.0 g
Cholesterol	**3 mg**
Sodium	**55 mg**
Potassium	**270 mg**
Total Carbohydrate	**4 g**
Dietary Fiber	1 g
Sugars	2 g
Protein	**4 g**
Phosphorus	**85 mg**

CHOICES/EXCHANGES

1 Nonstarchy Vegetable, 1/2 Fat

Main Dishes

Lemon Garlic Grilled Shrimp

This shrimp is marinated in a lemony garlic marinade, then skewered and cooked to perfection on the grill. Pair these shrimp with your favorite nonstarchy vegetable side and serve over brown rice.

INGREDIENTS

1/4 cup lemon juice
2 Tbsp olive oil
1/4 tsp red pepper flakes
2 cloves garlic, crushed
1 1/2 lb peeled, deveined raw shrimp*
24 wooden skewers

Prep Time: 5 minutes
Marinating Time: 30–60 minutes
Cook Time: 8 minutes
Serves: 6
Serving Size: 2 skewers

DIRECTIONS

1. In a small bowl, combine lemon juice, olive oil, red pepper flakes, and garlic and whisk to make marinade.
2. Place shrimp in a large resealable plastic bag and pour marinade over shrimp. Seal bag and let shrimp marinate in the refrigerator for at least 30 minutes (up to 60 minutes).
3. While shrimp are marinating, soak 24 skewers in water.
4. Remove bag of shrimp from the refrigerator and remove skewers from water. Take two skewers side by side and thread 5 shrimp onto them. (Using two skewers instead of one makes for easier turning on the grill.) Repeat for remaining skewers and shrimp to make a total of 12 skewers. Discard any remaining marinade.
5. Heat grill to medium heat and grill skewers about 4 minutes per side or until shrimp are opaque and pink. Remove from grill and enjoy!

*If possible, use fresh (never frozen) shrimp or shrimp that are free of preservatives [for example, shrimp that have not been treated with salt or STPP (sodium tripolyphosphate)].

BASIC NUTRITIONAL VALUES

Calories	**130**
Calories from Fat	30
Total Fat	**3.5 g**
Saturated Fat	0.5 g
Trans Fat	0.0 g
Cholesterol	**190 mg**
Sodium	**115 mg**
Potassium	**270 mg**
Total Carbohydrate	**1 g**
Dietary Fiber	0 g
Sugars	0 g
Protein	**24 g**
Phosphorus	**240 mg**

CHOICES/EXCHANGES

3 Lean Protein

Pan-Seared Scallops with Vegetable Ribbons

Here's an elegant dish for a special occasion. It's sure to impress, but it's also surprisingly easy to pull together!

INGREDIENTS

2 medium zucchini (6 oz each)
4 medium carrots
1 Tbsp plus 1 tsp olive oil, divided
1 lb scallops*
2 cloves garlic, minced
1 shallot, thinly sliced
1 cup white wine
2 tsp trans fat–free margarine
Freshly ground black pepper, to taste
5 Tbsp freshly grated Parmesan cheese

Prep Time: 15 minutes
Cook Time: 20 minutes
Serves: 5
Serving Size: 1 cup vegetable ribbons, about 3 oz scallops, and 1 Tbsp Parmesan

DIRECTIONS

1. Using a vegetable peeler, slice zucchini and carrots into "ribbons" and set aside. Note: If you have a spiralizer, you can use that to cut the zucchini and carrots.

2. In a large skillet, heat 1 Tbsp olive oil over medium-high heat. Add scallops to pan and sear for 3–5 minutes; then flip and sear for another 2–3 minutes until cooked through and slightly browned on both sides. Remove from pan and set aside in a covered bowl to keep warm.

3. Lower heat to medium and add remaining 1 tsp olive oil to the pan, then add garlic and shallot and sauté for 2 minutes.

4. Pour white wine in pan and scrape browned bits from the bottom of pan to deglaze it. Let wine simmer for 3 minutes until reduced by half, then add margarine and pepper. Add vegetable ribbons to wine sauce and toss to coat. Cover pan and allow vegetables to cook for 5 minutes.

5. To serve, place 1 cup of vegetables in bowl with about 3 oz scallops; then top with 1 Tbsp Parmesan cheese.

*If possible, use fresh (never frozen) scallops or scallops that are free of preservatives [for example, scallops that have not been treated with salt or STPP (sodium tripolyphosphate)].

BASIC NUTRITIONAL VALUES

Calories	180
Calories from Fat	60
Total Fat	**7.0 g**
Saturated Fat	1.8 g
Trans Fat	0.0 g
Cholesterol	**25 mg**
Sodium	**270 mg**
Potassium	**550 mg**
Total Carbohydrate	**12 g**
Dietary Fiber	2 g
Sugars	4 g
Protein	**15 g**
Phosphorus	**325 mg**

CHOICES/EXCHANGES

2 Nonstarchy Vegetable, 2 Lean Protein, 1 Fat

Pecan-Crusted Pork Tenderloin with Apples and Onions

This recipe comes together quickly, with the perfect combination of sweet and savory ingredients. It's sure to please!

Prep Time: 10 minutes
Cook Time: 30 minutes
Serves: 6
Serving Size: 2 slices pork (4 oz) and 3 Tbsp apple/onion mixture

INGREDIENTS

1 Tbsp chopped sage
1 clove garlic, minced
1/4 tsp salt
Freshly ground black pepper, to taste
5 tsp olive oil, divided
1/4 cup chopped pecans
1 1/2 lb pork tenderloin
1 medium onion, sliced
1 Braeburn apple, sliced (about 1/2-inch-thick slices)

DIRECTIONS

1. Preheat oven to 425°F.
2. In a small bowl, combine sage, garlic, salt, pepper, 1 tsp olive oil, and pecans. Mix well.
3. Pat pork tenderloin dry and brush with 2 tsp olive oil. Top with a layer of pecan mixture and set aside.
4. Heat remaining 2 tsp olive oil in a large ovenproof skillet over medium heat. Add onion and apples and sauté for 5 minutes; then place pork tenderloin in the same pan and cook for 20–25 minutes in the oven or until internal temperature reaches 145°F.
5. To serve, cut pork into 12 equal slices and top with apple and onion mixture.

BASIC NUTRITIONAL VALUES

Calories	**210**
Calories from Fat	90
Total Fat	**10.0 g**
Saturated Fat	1.8 g
Trans Fat	0.0 g
Cholesterol	**60 mg**
Sodium	**140 mg**
Potassium	**430 mg**
Total Carbohydrate	**6 g**
Dietary Fiber	1 g
Sugars	4 g
Protein	**23 g**
Phosphorus	**220 mg**

CHOICES/EXCHANGES

1/2 Carbohydrate, 3 Lean Protein, 1 Fat

Chicken Pesto Pasta Salad

This pasta salad tastes great hot or cold. Eat it fresh off the stove or over greens the day after cooking for lunch.

INGREDIENTS

6 oz dry whole-wheat rotini pasta
1/2 cup nonfat, plain Greek yogurt
2 Tbsp store-bought pesto
1/2 tsp lemon zest
Juice of 1/2 lemon
1 cup shredded rotisserie or other precooked chicken
1/3 cup diced red onion
1 cup diced yellow pepper
2 cups cherry tomatoes, sliced
1/3 cup crumbled feta cheese
1/3 cup chopped basil

Prep Time: 15 minutes
Cook Time: 10 minutes
Serves: 7
Serving Size: 1 cup

DIRECTIONS

1. Prepare pasta according to package instructions, omitting any added salt.
2. In a small mixing bowl, combine yogurt, pesto, lemon zest, and lemon juice. Mix well and set aside.
3. Once cooked, drain pasta and place in a large bowl. Add chicken, red onion, yellow pepper, and tomatoes.
4. Pour yogurt-pesto mixture over top and toss lightly to coat pasta salad. Stir in feta cheese and basil.

BASIC NUTRITIONAL VALUES

Calories	**180**
Calories from Fat	40
Total Fat	**4.5 g**
Saturated Fat	1.7 g
Trans Fat	0.1 g
Cholesterol	**30 mg**
Sodium	**210 mg**
Potassium	**280 mg**
Total Carbohydrate	**23 g**
Dietary Fiber	4 g
Sugars	3 g
Protein	**13 g**
Phosphorus	**165 mg**

CHOICES/EXCHANGES

1 Starch, 1 Nonstarchy Vegetable,
1 Lean Protein, 1/2 Fat

Pineapple Chile Chicken

This sweet and spicy chicken dish is perfect for a summer evening when served with fresh mango slices and Tropical Quinoa (page 138).

INGREDIENTS

1 cup pineapple juice*
1 Tbsp minced fresh ginger
1 Tbsp sliced green onion
1/2 tsp ancho chile powder
1/8 tsp salt
1 lb boneless skinless chicken breast, cut into 8 equal slices

Prep Time: 15 minutes
Marinating Time: At least 1 hour
Cook Time: 8 minutes
Serves: 4
Serving Size: 2 slices chicken (about 3 oz)

DIRECTIONS

1. In a large bowl, mix pineapple juice, ginger, green onion, ancho chile powder, and salt together.
2. Add sliced chicken to marinade and let sit, covered, in the refrigerator for at least 1 hour.
3. Remove chicken from marinade, reserving marinade.
4. Heat a skillet to medium-high heat and add 1/4 cup marinade. Place chicken in skillet and cook for 4 minutes on each side until chicken is golden brown and reaches an internal temperature of 160°F.
5. Discard unused marinade and enjoy!

*You can use pineapple juice reserved from the Tropical Quinoa recipe (page 138) in this recipe.

BASIC NUTRITIONAL VALUES

Calories	140
Calories from Fat	25
Total Fat	**3.0 g**
Saturated Fat	0.8 g
Trans Fat	0.0 g
Cholesterol	**65 mg**
Sodium	**95 mg**
Potassium	**240 mg**
Total Carbohydrate	**4 g**
Dietary Fiber	0 g
Sugars	3 g
Protein	**24 g**
Phosphorus	**175 mg**

CHOICES/EXCHANGES

3 Lean Protein

Salmon with Mango and Tomato Salsa

Mango and other fruit can add a slight sweetness to any salsa. It works particularly well with this slightly spicy salmon dish.

INGREDIENTS

Nonstick cooking spray
1 Tbsp chili powder
1 Tbsp cumin
1/4 tsp garlic powder
1/4 tsp cinnamon
1/4 tsp salt
1 1/2 lb salmon, cut into 6 (4-oz) fillets
1 1/2 cups diced mango
1 1/2 cups diced tomatoes
1/2 cup chopped cilantro
Juice of 1 lemon, divided

Prep Time: 15 minutes
Cook Time: 10 minutes
Serves: 6
Serving Size: 1 salmon fillet (4 oz) and 1/2 cup salsa

DIRECTIONS

1. Preheat oven to 425°F. Spray a shallow baking pan with cooking spray.
2. In a small bowl, combine chili powder, cumin, garlic powder, cinnamon, and salt. Mix and set aside.
3. Place salmon in shallow baking pan, then sprinkle spice mixture evenly over salmon fillets.
4. Place salmon in the oven and cook for 10 minutes or until cooked through.
5. While salmon is cooking, combine mango, tomatoes, cilantro, and half of the lemon juice in a medium bowl.
6. Remove salmon from oven and spritz with remaining lemon juice. Serve each fillet with 1/2 cup salsa.

BASIC NUTRITIONAL VALUES

Calories	**220**
Calories from Fat	80
Total Fat	**9.0 g**
Saturated Fat	1.9 g
Trans Fat	0.0 g
Cholesterol	**60 mg**
Sodium	**190 mg**
Potassium	**640 mg**
Total Carbohydrate	**10 g**
Dietary Fiber	2 g
Sugars	8 g
Protein	**23 g**
Phosphorus	**320 mg**

CHOICES/EXCHANGES

1/2 Fruit, 1 Nonstarchy Vegetable, 3 Lean Protein

Sesame Ginger Fried Tofu with Broccoli

Fried tofu is a great way to incorporate more plant-based proteins into your meals. It takes a little practice to cook but is worth the effort!

INGREDIENTS

1 (14-oz) package firm tofu
1/2 cup orange juice
1/4 cup diced fresh ginger
1/4 tsp dried ginger
1/4 cup chopped green onions (1 small bunch)
1 Tbsp reduced-sodium soy sauce
1 Tbsp sesame oil
1 Tbsp canola oil
1 Tbsp sesame seeds
4 cups fresh broccoli florets

Prep Time: 20 minutes
Marinating Time: At least 1 hour
Cook Time: 10 minutes
Serves: 4
Serving Size: 3 slices tofu and about 1 cup broccoli

DIRECTIONS

1. Slice block of tofu into 12 slices (cut down the middle and then cut 6 pieces on each side).
2. Place tofu slices on several layers of paper towels. Cover with paper towels and set a heavy pan on top to press out excess liquid.
3. In a large bowl, mix together orange juice, fresh ginger, dried ginger, green onions, soy sauce, and sesame oil.

4. Add the slices of tofu to bowl and marinate for at least 1 hour in the refrigerator. Note: Marinating for several hours is better to allow tofu to absorb more flavor.

5. Heat canola oil in a skillet over medium heat. Place tofu on skillet (reserve marinade) and fry for 4 minutes. Flip and fry for 4 more minutes until brown on each side. Adjust heat as needed to prevent burning.

6. Remove tofu from skillet, sprinkle with sesame seeds, and cover with foil to keep warm.

7. Add broccoli and remaining marinade, including fresh ginger and green onions, into the skillet. Sauté the broccoli over low heat for 5 minutes or until tender. Marinade will caramelize a bit on the broccoli. Serve broccoli with tofu and enjoy!

BASIC NUTRITIONAL VALUES

Calories	190
Calories from Fat	120
Total Fat	**13.0 g**
Saturated Fat	1.8 g
Trans Fat	0.0 g
Cholesterol	**0 mg**
Sodium	**170 mg**
Potassium	**500 mg**
Total Carbohydrate	**11 g**
Dietary Fiber	4 g
Sugars	5 g
Protein	**11 g**
Phosphorus	**195 mg**

CHOICES/EXCHANGES

1/2 Carbohydrate, 1 Nonstarchy Vegetable, 1 Medium-Fat Protein, 1 1/2 Fat

Shrimp Fried Cauliflower Rice

Here's a unique spin on fried rice with fewer carbs per serving and filling protein from the shrimp!

INGREDIENTS

1 Tbsp olive oil, divided
16 oz peeled, deveined raw shrimp*
4 green onions, sliced
1 cup chopped carrots
1 Tbsp minced fresh ginger
15 oz (about 4 cups) riced cauliflower
2 tsp reduced-sodium soy sauce
Juice of 1 lime

Prep Time: 10 minutes
Cook Time: 20 minutes
Serves: 4
Serving Size: 1 cup

DIRECTIONS

1. Heat 1 tsp olive oil in a small skillet over medium-high heat. Add shrimp and cook for 3–5 minutes until it turns pink and opaque. Remove from skillet and set aside.
2. In a large skillet, heat remaining 2 tsp olive oil over medium heat. Add green onions and carrots and cook for 5 minutes. Add ginger and cook for an additional 2 minutes.
3. Add cauliflower rice and soy sauce and cook for an additional 5–7 minutes or until cooked through and cauliflower begins to brown.
4. Stir in shrimp and top with lime juice.

*If possible, use fresh (never frozen) shrimp or shrimp that are free of preservatives [for example, shrimp that have not been treated with salt or STPP (sodium tripolyphosphate)].

Tip: You can find bags of fresh or frozen cauliflower rice in many grocery stores.

BASIC NUTRITIONAL VALUES

Calories	**180**
Calories from Fat	35
Total Fat	**4.0 g**
Saturated Fat	0.7 g
Trans Fat	0.0 g
Cholesterol	**190 mg**
Sodium	**260 mg**
Potassium	**740 mg**
Total Carbohydrate	**11 g**
Dietary Fiber	3 g
Sugars	4 g
Protein	**27 g**
Phosphorus	**305 mg**

CHOICES/EXCHANGES

2 Nonstarchy Vegetable,
3 Lean Protein

Simple Roasted Salmon

Are you intimidated when it comes to cooking fish for dinner? Don't be! Here is a quick and simple salmon recipe that's high in protein and healthy fats.

INGREDIENTS

Nonstick cooking spray
4 fresh salmon fillets (about 4 oz each)
1 Tbsp olive oil
1 tsp dried dill
1/4 tsp freshly ground black pepper
2 tsp lemon juice

Prep Time: 5 minutes
Cook Time: 12 minutes
Serves: 4
Serving Size: 1 salmon fillet (about 4 oz)

DIRECTIONS

1. Preheat oven to 425°F and coat a glass baking dish with cooking spray.
2. Lay the salmon fillets in the baking dish and brush the top of each fillet with the olive oil.
3. Sprinkle dill and pepper evenly over each fillet and roast in the oven for 10–12 minutes, or until the fish is opaque and flakes when touched with a fork.
4. Remove fish from the oven, pour lemon juice evenly over each fillet, and serve immediately.

BASIC NUTRITIONAL VALUES

Calories	**200**
Calories from Fat	110
Total Fat	**12.0 g**
Saturated Fat	2.3 g
Trans Fat	0.0 g
Cholesterol	**60 mg**
Sodium	**75 mg**
Potassium	**410 mg**
Total Carbohydrate	**0 g**
Dietary Fiber	0 g
Sugars	0 g
Protein	**22 g**
Phosphorus	**295 mg**

CHOICES/EXCHANGES

3 Lean Protein, 1 Fat

Slow-Cooker Beef Tacos

Enjoy these delicious slow-cooker tacos any night of the week. This dish can also be easily frozen to enjoy at a later date!

INGREDIENTS

1/2 cup reduced-sodium beef broth
2 Tbsp tomato paste
1 Tbsp cumin
2 tsp chili powder
1 Tbsp olive oil
2 1/4 lb extra-lean beef roast (such as eye of round roast)
1 large onion, sliced
2 poblano peppers, sliced
12 (6-inch) corn tortillas
1 1/2 cups low-sodium pico de gallo
6 Tbsp crumbled feta cheese, divided

Prep Time: 30 minutes
Cook Time: 6 hours (may vary based on your slow cooker)
Serves: 12
Serving Size: 1 taco

DIRECTIONS

1. In a small mixing bowl, whisk together broth, tomato paste, cumin, and chili powder. Set aside.

2. Heat olive oil over medium-high heat in a sauté pan; then sear each side of the beef roast for about 4 minutes per side or until slightly browned.

3. Place onion and peppers in a layer at the bottom of the slow cooker. Place seared beef roast over the vegetables and pour broth mixture over the roast. Cover and cook on

low for 6 hours or until beef is tender and cooked through (to an internal temperature of least 145°F).

4. Remove beef from slow cooker and shred; then add it back to the liquid and veggies and stir to combine.

5. To make one taco, place one tortilla on a plate and top with 1/3 cup beef and veggies, 2 Tbsp pico de gallo, and 1/2 Tbsp feta cheese.

Tip: Like lots of toppings on your tacos? Other nutritious toppings that you can add include shredded cabbage or a dollop of nonfat, plain Greek yogurt!

BASIC NUTRITIONAL VALUES

Calories	210
Calories from Fat	50
Total Fat	**6.0 g**
Saturated Fat	1.9 g
Trans Fat	0.0 g
Cholesterol	**40 mg**
Sodium	**130 mg**
Potassium	**360 mg**
Total Carbohydrate	**17 g**
Dietary Fiber	2 g
Sugars	3 g
Protein	**23 g**
Phosphorus	**245 mg**

CHOICES/EXCHANGES

1 Starch, 1 Nonstarchy Vegetable, 2 Lean Protein, 1/2 Fat

Spicy Slow-Cooker Chicken

The tomatoes in this dish keep the chicken moist and create a flavorful sauce. Try pairing this dish with Pine Nut Olive Couscous (page 125).

INGREDIENTS

2 lb boneless, skinless chicken breasts
2 (14.5-oz) cans diced tomatoes, undrained
2 Tbsp capers
1 large onion, chopped (1 1/2 cups)
1 tsp dried basil
1/4 tsp red pepper flakes

Prep Time: 10 minutes
Cook Time: 3 1/2 hours (on low)
Serves: 8
Serving Size: About 3/4 cup sauce and 3 oz chicken

DIRECTIONS

1. Add all ingredients to a slow cooker.
2. Cook on low heat for 3 1/2 hours.
3. Remove chicken and slice before serving. Top each serving of chicken with 3/4 cup sauce.

BASIC NUTRITIONAL VALUES

Calories	160
Calories from Fat	25
Total Fat	**3.0 g**
Saturated Fat	0.8 g
Trans Fat	0.0 g
Cholesterol	**65 mg**
Sodium	**260 mg**
Potassium	**430 mg**
Total Carbohydrate	**7 g**
Dietary Fiber	2 g
Sugars	4 g
Protein	**25 g**
Phosphorus	**200 mg**

CHOICES/EXCHANGES

1 Nonstarchy Vegetable,
3 Lean Protein

Spinach and Turkey Meatballs

Serve up these tender meatballs for a fun twist on Italian night!

INGREDIENTS

16 oz 93%-lean ground turkey
1 egg
3 Tbsp freshly grated Parmesan cheese
2 cloves garlic, crushed
1/2 cup whole-wheat bread crumbs
2 tsp dried basil
Freshly ground black pepper, to taste
10 oz chopped steamed spinach
Nonstick cooking spray

Prep Time: 20 minutes
Cook Time: 20 minutes
Serves: 6
Serving Size: 4 meatballs

DIRECTIONS

1. Preheat oven to 400°F.
2. Place all ingredients, except cooking spray, in a large mixing bowl and mix together thoroughly.
3. Roll into 24 golf ball–sized meatballs (about 2 Tbsp each).
4. Spray a 9 × 13-inch baking pan with cooking spray and place meatballs in the pan. Bake in the oven for 20 minutes.
5. Remove meatballs from oven and serve hot. Enjoy with 3/4 cup whole-wheat pasta and 1/3 cup of your favorite chunky tomato sauce if desired.

BASIC NUTRITIONAL VALUES

Calories	**180**
Calories from Fat	60
Total Fat	**7.0 g**
Saturated Fat	2.3 g
Trans Fat	0.1 g
Cholesterol	**90 mg**
Sodium	**140 mg**
Potassium	**320 mg**
Total Carbohydrate	**8 g**
Dietary Fiber	2 g
Sugars	1 g
Protein	**19 g**
Phosphorus	**205 mg**

CHOICES/EXCHANGES

1/2 Starch, 2 Lean Protein, 1 Fat

Tilapia with Pesto Vinaigrette and Tomatoes

Try this zesty fish entrée paired with a nice green salad and small piece of garlic bread.

INGREDIENTS

1 lb tilapia fillets
1/3 cup Pesto Vinaigrette (page 21)
2 cups grape tomatoes, halved
1 tsp olive oil
1/8 tsp salt
Freshly ground black pepper, to taste
Nonstick cooking spray
1/4 cup chopped basil (for garnish)

Prep Time: 5 minutes
Marinating Time: 30 minutes
Cook Time: 10 minutes
Serves: 4
Serving Size: 4 oz tilapia and 1/3 cup of tomatoes/sauce

DIRECTIONS

1. Place tilapia fillets and Pesto Vinaigrette in a large resealable plastic bag. Seal the bag and let fish marinate in the refrigerator for 30 minutes.
2. In a medium bowl, toss tomatoes, olive oil, salt, and pepper together.
3. Spray a large skillet with cooking spray and heat over medium-high heat. Pour marinated fish, excess marinade, and tomatoes into skillet and toss tomatoes lightly to coat them with marinade. Cook fish on one side for 4–5 minutes, then flip and cook for an additional 2–3 minutes or until cooked through. Serve hot.

BASIC NUTRITIONAL VALUES

Calories	**180**
Calories from Fat	70
Total Fat	**8.0 g**
Saturated Fat	1.7 g
Trans Fat	0.0 g
Cholesterol	**50 mg**
Sodium	**170 mg**
Potassium	**530 mg**
Total Carbohydrate	**4 g**
Dietary Fiber	1 g
Sugars	2 g
Protein	**23 g**
Phosphorus	**195 mg**

CHOICES/EXCHANGES

3 Lean Protein, 1 Fat

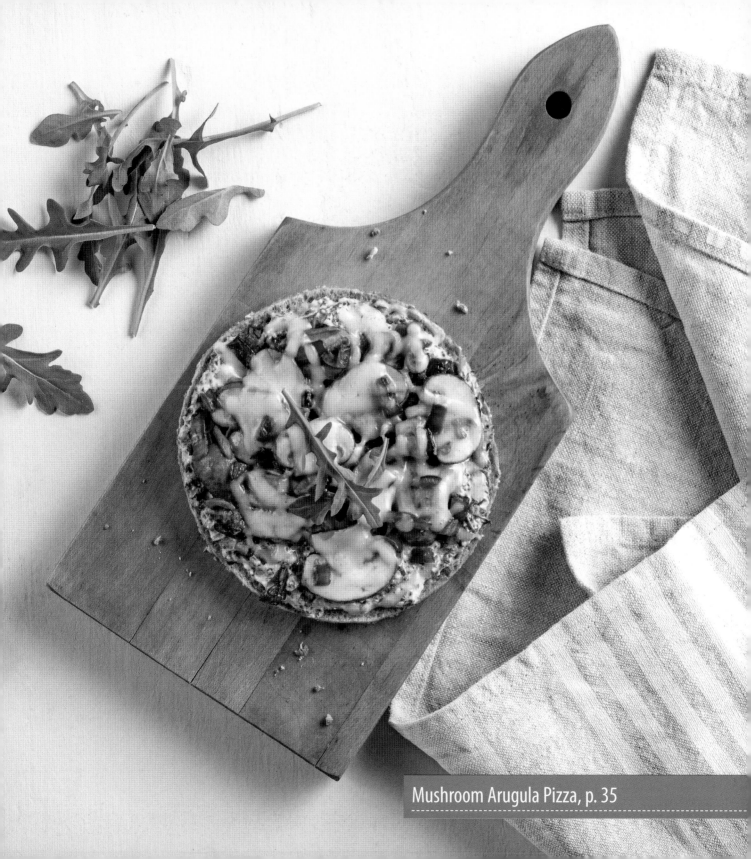

Mushroom Arugula Pizza, p. 35

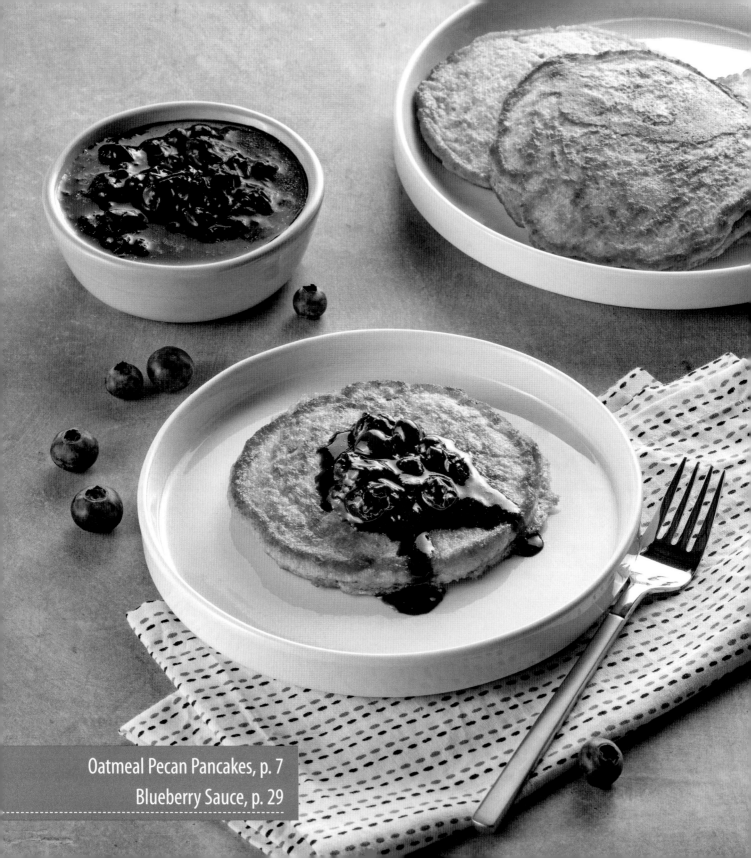

Oatmeal Pecan Pancakes, p. 7
Blueberry Sauce, p. 29

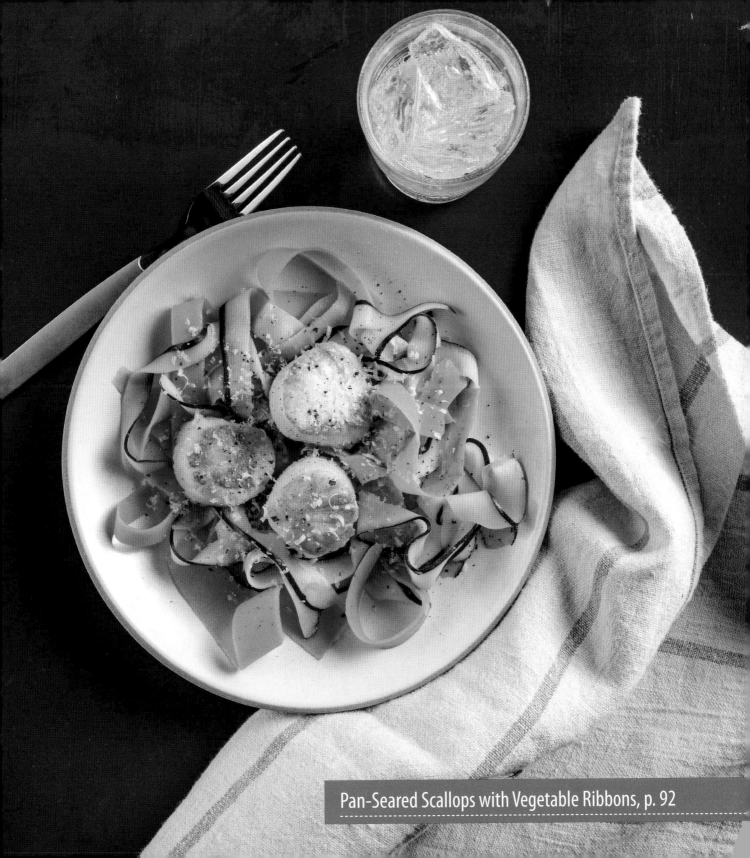

Pan-Seared Scallops with Vegetable Ribbons, p. 92

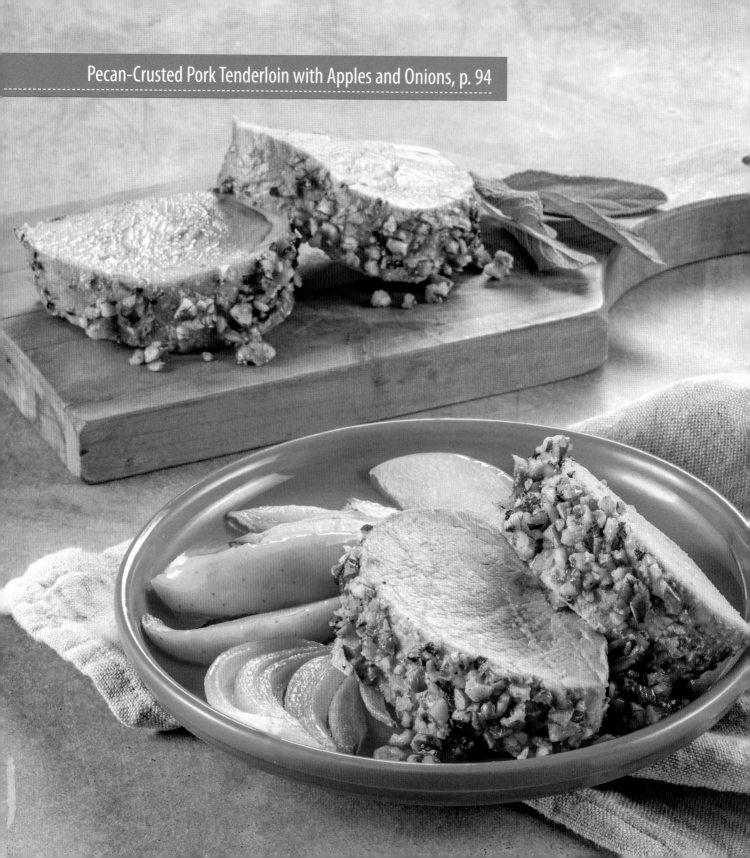

Pecan-Crusted Pork Tenderloin with Apples and Onions, p. 94

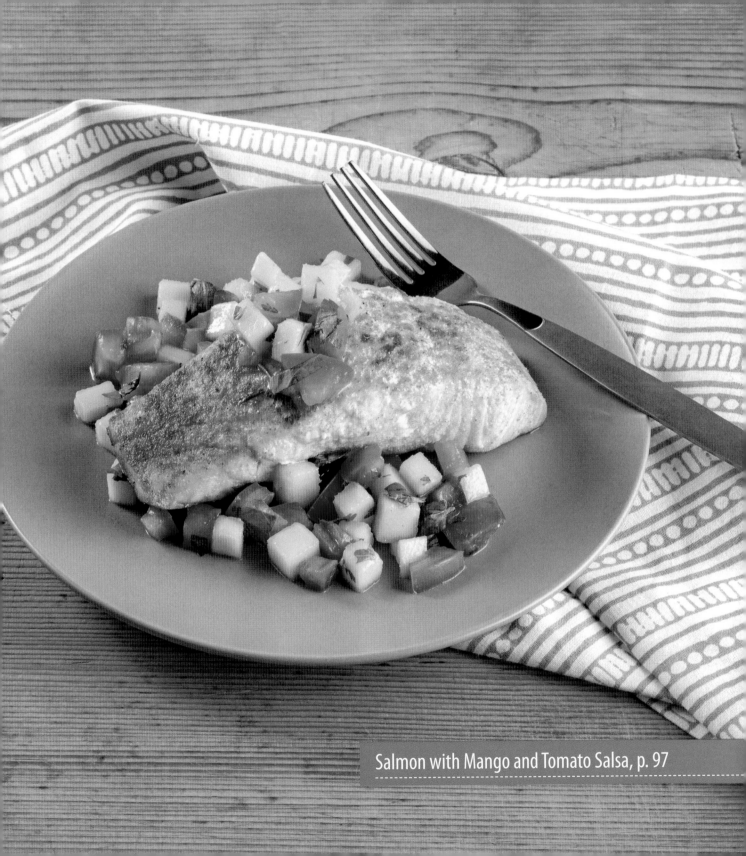

Salmon with Mango and Tomato Salsa, p. 97

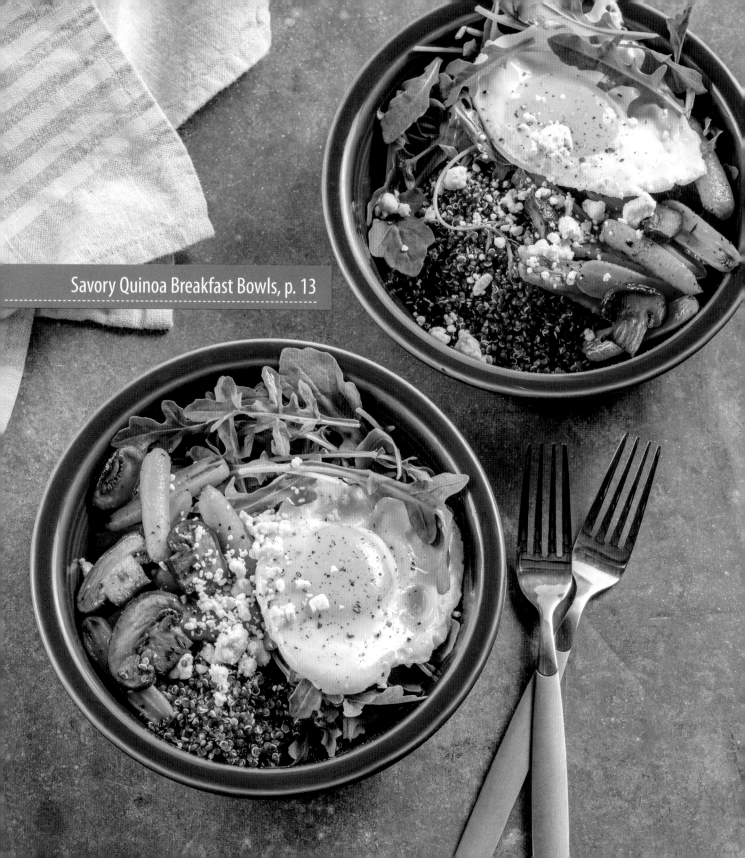

Savory Quinoa Breakfast Bowls, p. 13

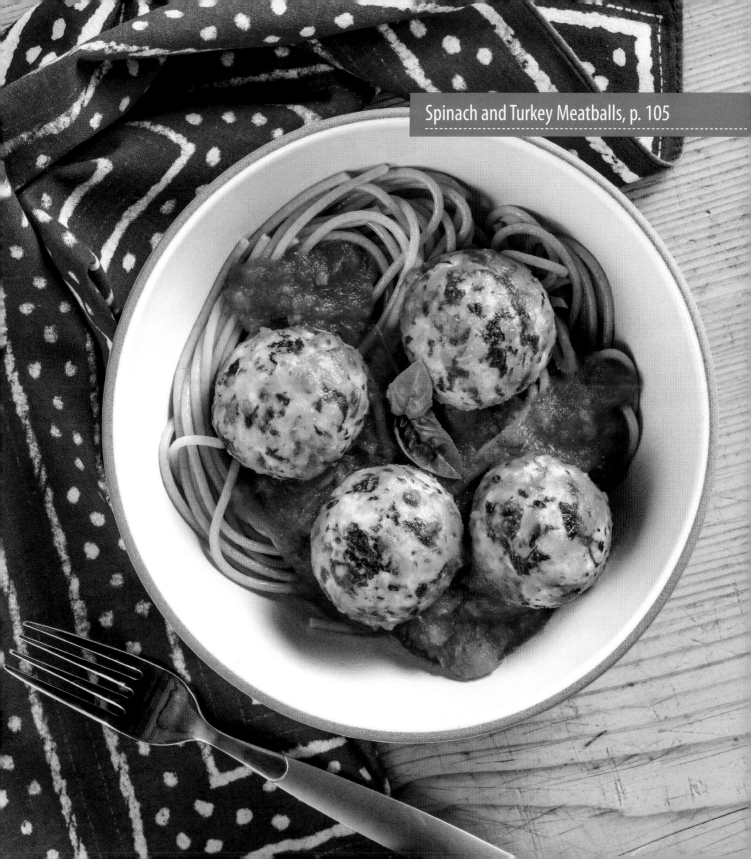

Spinach and Turkey Meatballs, p. 105

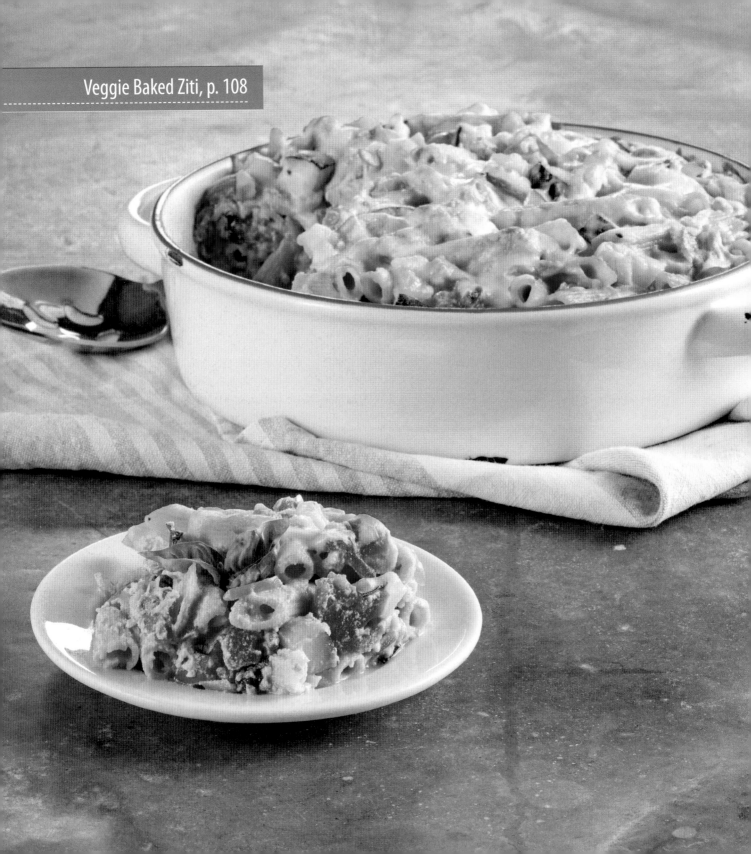

Veggie Baked Ziti, p. 108

Turkey Tacos

Lean ground turkey makes a great base for a delicious taco meal. This recipe has a spicy kick that can be adjusted by adding more or less jalapeño.

INGREDIENTS

2 tsp olive oil
1/2 red onion, diced
2 Tbsp finely diced jalapeño
16 oz 93%-lean ground turkey
1 large clove garlic, minced
1 Tbsp cumin
1 Tbsp chili powder
1/2 tsp smoked paprika
2 Tbsp water
6 (6-inch) corn tortillas
1 large (8-oz) avocado, diced
6 Tbsp nonfat, plain Greek yogurt
6 Tbsp no-salt-added pico de gallo

Prep Time: 10 minutes
Cook Time: 5 minutes
Serves: 6
Serving Size: 1 taco

DIRECTIONS

1. In a large skillet, heat olive oil over medium-high heat.
2. Add onion and jalapeño to skillet and cook for 2 minutes. Add turkey and cook until turkey is browned and vegetables are cooked through, about 5–7 minutes. Add garlic and cumin and cook for 30 seconds.
3. Lower heat and add chili powder, smoked paprika, and water and mix thoroughly.
4. Fill each tortilla with 1/2 cup turkey mixture, plus about 2 Tbsp diced avocado, 1 Tbsp Greek yogurt, and 1 Tbsp pico de gallo.

BASIC NUTRITIONAL VALUES

Calories	**260**
Calories from Fat	110
Total Fat	**12.0 g**
Saturated Fat	2.6 g
Trans Fat	0.1 g
Cholesterol	**60 mg**
Sodium	**80 mg**
Potassium	**460 mg**
Total Carbohydrate	**19 g**
Dietary Fiber	4 g
Sugars	2 g
Protein	**19 g**
Phosphorus	**275 mg**

CHOICES/EXCHANGES

1 Starch, 1 Nonstarchy Vegetable,
2 Lean Protein, 1 1/2 Fat

Veggie Baked Ziti

Enjoy a vegetarian twist on this favorite pasta dish.

INGREDIENTS

8 oz dry whole-wheat ziti
2 tsp olive oil
1 cup chopped onion
2 cups sliced zucchini
1 cup chopped red pepper
1 cup fat-free ricotta cheese
1 egg
1/4 cup shredded Parmesan cheese
Freshly ground black pepper, to taste
1 (14.5-oz) can no-salt-added diced tomatoes
1/2 cup chopped fresh basil
Nonstick cooking spray
2/3 cup part-skim mozzarella

Prep Time: 30 minutes
Cook Time: 30 minutes
Serves: 12
Serving Size:
1 (3 1/4 × 3-inch) piece

DIRECTIONS

1. Prepare pasta according to package instructions, omitting any added salt or fat. Preheat oven to 375°F.

2. Heat olive oil in a large skillet over medium heat. Add onion and sauté for 4 minutes. Then add zucchini and red pepper and sauté for another 5–7 minutes or until veggies are cooked through.

3. While veggies are cooking, whisk together ricotta, egg, Parmesan, and pepper in a small bowl.

4. Add diced tomatoes to cooked veggie mixture and heat through. Stir in basil, pasta, and ricotta mixture.

5. Spray a 9 × 13-inch baking dish with cooking spray, pour in ziti mixture, and sprinkle mozzarella evenly over top. Bake for 25 minutes and serve immediately.

BASIC NUTRITIONAL VALUES

Calories	130
Calories from Fat	25
Total Fat	**3.0 g**
Saturated Fat	1.1 g
Trans Fat	0.0 g
Cholesterol	**25 mg**
Sodium	**90 mg**
Potassium	**230 mg**
Total Carbohydrate	**19 g**
Dietary Fiber	3 g
Sugars	4 g
Protein	**9 g**
Phosphorus	**150 mg**

CHOICES/EXCHANGES

1 Starch, 1 Nonstarchy Vegetable, 1/2 Fat

Greek Yogurt–Marinated Grilled Chicken

A simple marinade using the versatile ingredient Greek yogurt makes this tender, flavor-packed chicken dish a crowd-pleaser at dinnertime!

INGREDIENTS

1 3/4 lb boneless, skinless chicken breasts
2/3 cup nonfat, plain Greek yogurt
1 Tbsp olive oil
Zest and juice of 1 lemon
1 clove garlic, crushed or minced
1 tsp dried oregano
1/4 tsp red pepper flakes

DIRECTIONS

1. Place chicken breasts in a large, gallon-size resealable plastic bag. Set aside.
2. In a small mixing bowl, combine the remaining ingredients to make the marinade. Pour marinade over chicken to coat. Then squeeze any extra air out of the bag and seal it.
3. Marinate chicken in the refrigerator for at least 1 hour or overnight.
4. Once finished marinating, discard any unabsorbed marinade, and cook chicken in the oven at 400°F for 35–40 minutes, or until internal temperature reaches 165°F.

Prep Time: 10 minutes
Marinating Time: At least 1 hour or overnight
Cook Time: 40 minutes
Serves: 6
Serving Size: About 4 oz chicken

BASIC NUTRITIONAL VALUES

Calories	**170**
Calories from Fat	40
Total Fat	**4.5 g**
Saturated Fat	1.1 g
Trans Fat	0.0 g
Cholesterol	**75 mg**
Sodium	**70 mg**
Potassium	**250 mg**
Total Carbohydrate	**1 g**
Dietary Fiber	0 g
Sugars	1 g
Protein	**29 g**
Phosphorus	**220 mg**

CHOICES/EXCHANGES

4 Lean Protein

Chicken Stroganoff

In the mood for a hearty, comforting dish? This lightened-up Chicken Stroganoff delivers just that!

INGREDIENTS

4 oz dry whole-wheat egg noodles
2 tsp olive oil
1/2 onion, chopped
16 oz mushrooms, sliced
1 1/4 lb chicken breast, cut into bite-size pieces
2 cloves garlic, minced
1 Tbsp chopped thyme
Freshly ground black pepper, to taste
2 Tbsp all-purpose flour
1 1/4 cups reduced-sodium chicken broth
2 Tbsp marsala wine
1 cup nonfat, plain Greek yogurt

Prep Time: 15 minutes
Cook Time: 20 minutes
Serves: 7
Serving Size: 1 cup

DIRECTIONS

1. Prepare egg noodles according to package instructions, omitting any added salt.

2. While noodles are cooking, heat olive oil in a large skillet over medium-high heat. Add onions and mushrooms and sauté for 7 minutes, stirring occasionally.

3. Push mushrooms and onions to the side of the pan and add chicken, garlic, thyme, and pepper to the center. Slowly mix ingredients together as chicken cooks for about 4–5 more minutes.

4. When most of the liquid in the pan has evaporated, add flour and mix to coat chicken and vegetables. Cook for 30 seconds, and then add broth and marsala wine. Let chicken mixture simmer, stirring occasionally, about 5 minutes or until liquid is reduced by half.

5. Remove pan from heat and stir in noodles and yogurt. Mix thoroughly and serve immediately.

BASIC NUTRITIONAL VALUES

Calories	**210**
Calories from Fat	35
Total Fat	**4.0 g**
Saturated Fat	0.9 g
Trans Fat	0.0 g
Cholesterol	**50 mg**
Sodium	**160 mg**
Potassium	**490 mg**
Total Carbohydrate	**18 g**
Dietary Fiber	3 g
Sugars	3 g
Protein	**25 g**
Phosphorus	**280 mg**

CHOICES/EXCHANGES

1 Starch, 1 Nonstarchy Vegetable, 3 Lean Protein

Chicken, Spinach, and Mushroom Enchiladas

These enchiladas make sneaking in more vegetables easy and delicious.

INGREDIENTS

Enchilada Sauce
1 (14.5-oz) can diced tomatoes
2 Tbsp tomato paste
2 tsp chili powder
2 tsp cumin

Enchiladas
1 Tbsp olive oil
1 cup diced onion
8 oz mushrooms
4 cups baby spinach
2 cups cooked chicken breast
2 light spreadable Swiss cheese wedges (such as Laughing Cow)
6 (6-inch) 100% whole-wheat tortillas
3/4 cup nonfat, plain Greek yogurt

Prep Time: 20 minutes
Cook Time: 30 minutes
Serves: 6
Serving Size: 1 enchilada

DIRECTIONS

1. Preheat oven to 375°F.

2. In a small saucepan, whisk together all Enchilada Sauce ingredients over low heat, and cook until heated through. Remove from heat and set aside.

3. In a large skillet, heat olive oil over medium heat. Add onion and mushrooms and cook for 5–7 minutes or until tender.

4. Add spinach and cook until wilted, about 2 minutes.

5. Add chicken and spreadable cheese wedges and mix until cheese has melted and coated the other ingredients.

6. Spread 1/4 cup sauce on the bottom of a 13 × 9-inch glass baking pan. Then, fill each tortilla with 1/2 cup chicken-and-vegetable filling and place in pan with seam side down. Once all enchiladas are in the pan, top each with 2 Tbsp of sauce and bake for 20 minutes.

7. Enjoy each enchilada topped with 2 Tbsp Greek yogurt.

BASIC NUTRITIONAL VALUES

Calories	**250**
Calories from Fat	70
Total Fat	**8.0 g**
Saturated Fat	2.6 g
Trans Fat	0.0 g
Cholesterol	**40 mg**
Sodium	**410 mg**
Potassium	**710 mg**
Total Carbohydrate	**23 g**
Dietary Fiber	5 g
Sugars	6 g
Protein	**24 g**
Phosphorus	**355 mg**

CHOICES/EXCHANGES

1 Starch, 2 Nonstarchy Vegetable, 2 Lean Protein, 1 Fat

Crispy Polenta with Veggies and White Beans

Here's a hearty vegetarian entrée that cooks in less than 30 minutes!

INGREDIENTS

1 Tbsp olive oil
15 oz prepared polenta, sliced into 10 thin
    slices
1/2 medium onion, diced (about 1 1/4 cups)
8 oz mushrooms, sliced
1 medium zucchini, sliced into half moons
1/4 tsp red pepper flakes
1 (15-oz) can reduced-sodium cannellini
    beans, drained and rinsed
1 (15-oz) can low-sodium diced tomatoes
5 Tbsp shredded Parmesan cheese

Prep Time: 10 minutes
Cook Time: 20 minutes
Serves: 5
Serving Size: 2 slices polenta,
1 cup veggie and bean
mixture, and 1 Tbsp cheese

DIRECTIONS

1. In a large skillet, heat olive oil over medium heat. Swirl pan to coat and add polenta slices. Sauté slices for approximately 5 minutes on each slide or until slightly golden and crispy. Remove polenta and set aside.

2. Add onion, mushrooms, and zucchini to the same pan where you cooked the polenta. Cook, stirring occasionally, for 8–10 minutes or until vegetables are cooked through and beginning to brown.

3. Add red pepper flakes, beans, and diced tomatoes and heat through for about 2 minutes.

4. Serve 1 cup of vegetable and bean mixture over 2 polenta slices and top with 1 Tbsp Parmesan cheese.

BASIC NUTRITIONAL VALUES

Calories	**200**
Calories from Fat	40
Total Fat	**4.5 g**
Saturated Fat	1.0 g
Trans Fat	0.0 g
Cholesterol	**0 mg**
Sodium	**280 mg**
Potassium	**700 mg**
Total Carbohydrate	**33 g**
Dietary Fiber	8 g
Sugars	6 g
Protein	**9 g**
Phosphorus	**190 mg**

CHOICES/EXCHANGES

1 1/2 Starch, 2 Nonstarchy Vegetable, 1/2 Fat

Slow-Cooker Roast Chicken and Root Vegetables

Come home to a delicious and healthful dinner *and* have leftovers the next day for lunch! You can add more herbs or even different ones to this dish for an extra kick.

INGREDIENTS

2 lb boneless, skinless chicken thighs (about 8–9 chicken thighs)
1 1/2 lb sweet potatoes
1 yellow onion
1 (16-oz) package baby carrots
1/2 tsp garlic powder
1 tsp rosemary
1 tsp poultry seasoning

DIRECTIONS

1. Wash chicken and pat dry. Set aside.
2. Chop sweet potatoes into 8 chunks and slice onion.
3. In the bottom of a slow cooker, layer potatoes, onion, and carrots, in that order.
4. Layer chicken on top of carrots.
5. In a small bowl, mix together garlic powder, rosemary, and poultry seasoning. Sprinkle spices over chicken.
6. Cook on low heat for 5–6 hours.

Prep Time: 10 minutes
Cook Time: 5–6 hours (on low)
Serves: 8
Serving Size: 1 chicken thigh (about 3 oz), 1 piece sweet potato, and 6 carrots

BASIC NUTRITIONAL VALUES

Calories	**240**
Calories from Fat	60
Total Fat	**7.0 g**
Saturated Fat	1.8 g
Trans Fat	0.0 g
Cholesterol	**105 mg**
Sodium	**150 mg**
Potassium	**710 mg**
Total Carbohydrate	**25 g**
Dietary Fiber	5 g
Sugars	7 g
Protein	**20 g**
Phosphorus	**230 mg**

CHOICES/EXCHANGES

1 Starch, 2 Nonstarchy Vegetable,
2 Lean Protein, 1/2 Fat

Honey Lime Chicken

Leftovers from this tangy and slightly sweet chicken can be used to make a quick wrap for lunch the next day.

INGREDIENTS

1/3 cup lime juice
2 cloves garlic
1 Tbsp olive oil
1 Tbsp honey
1/4 cup chopped green onions
1/2 cup chopped fresh cilantro
1/4 tsp salt
1 lb boneless, skinless chicken breast (4 small breasts)

Prep Time: 10 minutes
Marinating Time: At least 1 hour
Cook Time: 20 minutes
Serves: 4
Serving Size: 1 small chicken breast

DIRECTIONS

1. In a large bowl, mix together lime juice, garlic, olive oil, honey, green onions, cilantro, and salt.
2. Add chicken breasts to large resealable plastic bag.
3. Add marinade to the bag and lay flat in the refrigerator for at least 1 hour. Note: The longer the chicken is left to marinate, the more flavorful it will become.
4. Remove chicken from marinade and discard marinade.
5. Grill chicken to an internal temperature of 165°F.

BASIC NUTRITIONAL VALUES

Calories	**160**
Calories from Fat	45
Total Fat	**5.0 g**
Saturated Fat	1.1 g
Trans Fat	0.0 g
Cholesterol	**65 mg**
Sodium	**160 mg**
Potassium	**240 mg**
Total Carbohydrate	**5 g**
Dietary Fiber	0 g
Sugars	3 g
Protein	**24 g**
Phosphorus	**180 mg**

CHOICES/EXCHANGES

1/2 Carbohydrate,
3 Lean Protein

Eggplant, Quinoa, and Turkey Meat Loaf

Look no further for a way to sneak whole grains and nonstarchy vegetables into a meal. The eggplant in this dish helps absorb excess liquid and keeps the meat loaf moist. Try using other vegetables like shredded carrots or zucchini in this recipe if you want to experiment.

INGREDIENTS

1/2 cup dry tricolor quinoa
1/2 cup chopped onion
1/2 cup peeled, diced eggplant
1 clove garlic, crushed
1 tsp olive oil
1 lb ground turkey breast
1 egg
1 tsp hot sauce (such as Tabasco) or other chile sauce
1 tsp reduced-sodium Worcestershire sauce
1 Tbsp dried parsley
1/2 tsp dried thyme
1 tsp dried oregano
1 (6-oz) can tomato paste, divided
1/3 cup diced tomatoes, drained
Fresh ground black pepper, to taste

Prep Time: 20 minutes
Cook Time: 1 hour
Serves: 6
Serving Size: 1 slice

DIRECTIONS

1. Cook quinoa according to package instructions, omitting any added salt.
2. While quinoa is simmering, sauté onion, eggplant, and garlic in olive oil over medium heat for about 5 minutes.
3. In a large bowl, mix cooked quinoa, turkey, egg, hot sauce, Worcestershire sauce, parsley, thyme, oregano, 1/2 can tomato paste, and eggplant mixture together until well combined.
4. Spread meat loaf mixture evenly in a loaf pan.

5. In a separate bowl, mix diced tomatoes and remaining tomato paste together and spread evenly on top of meat loaf mixture. Top with pepper.

6. Bake at 350°F for 55 minutes or until internal temperature reaches 165°F.

7. Let meat loaf cool and cut into 6 slices.

BASIC NUTRITIONAL VALUES

Calories	200
Calories from Fat	35
Total Fat	**4.0 g**
Saturated Fat	0.9 g
Trans Fat	0.0 g
Cholesterol	**75 mg**
Sodium	**300 mg**
Potassium	**680 mg**
Total Carbohydrate	**18 g**
Dietary Fiber	3 g
Sugars	6 g
Protein	**24 g**
Phosphorus	**290 mg**

CHOICES/EXCHANGES

1/2 Starch, 2 Nonstarchy Vegetable, 2 Lean Protein, 1/2 Fat

Italian Stuffed Green Peppers

Using fat-free cottage cheese is a great alternative to ricotta cheese for all your Italian-style favorites.

INGREDIENTS

2 small (4-oz) green peppers
1/2 cup chopped onion
2 cloves garlic, crushed
1/2 tsp olive oil
1 cup fat-free cottage cheese
1 egg
2 cups frozen, chopped spinach, cooked in microwave and drained
1/4 cup freshly grated Parmesan cheese, divided
1 cup Simple Garlic Marinara Sauce (page 30)
Nonstick olive oil cooking spray

Prep Time: 20 minutes
Cook Time: 50 minutes
Serves: 4
Serving Size: 1/2 pepper with filling

DIRECTIONS

1. Preheat oven to 450°F.
2. Slice green peppers in half and remove seeds.
3. In a nonstick skillet, sauté onion and garlic in olive oil over medium heat.
4. Place cottage cheese and egg in a food processor or blender and blend until smooth. Add cooked spinach, 2 Tbsp Parmesan cheese, and onion and garlic mixture and process or blend until smooth.
5. Put 2 Tbsp of marinara sauce in each pepper half, covering the bottom. Add 1/3 cup cottage cheese mixture and top with another 2 Tbsp marinara sauce.
6. Sprinkle each pepper half with 1/2 Tbsp Parmesan cheese.
7. Spray bottom of a glass dish with oil cooking spray. Place filled green peppers in dish. Bake in the oven for 45 minutes.

BASIC NUTRITIONAL VALUES

Calories	**150**
Calories from Fat	40
Total Fat	**4.5 g**
Saturated Fat	1.5 g
Trans Fat	0.0 g
Cholesterol	**55 mg**
Sodium	**410 mg**
Potassium	**600 mg**
Total Carbohydrate	**17 g**
Dietary Fiber	5 g
Sugars	6 g
Protein	**13 g**
Phosphorus	**235 mg**

CHOICES/EXCHANGES

3 Nonstarchy Vegetable,
1 Lean Protein, 1/2 Fat

Side Dishes

Haricots Verts with Brown Rice, Pine Nuts, and Parmesan

For this recipe, use precooked brown rice and you'll have a nutritious side of whole grains and veggies ready in minutes!

Prep Time: 10 minutes
Cook Time: 7 minutes
Serves: 4
Serving Size: 1 cup

INGREDIENTS

3 cups trimmed, chopped haricots verts or French beans (1-inch pieces)
1 1/2 tsp olive oil
1 large shallot, thinly sliced
1 cup cooked brown rice (prepared without salt)
2 Tbsp shredded Parmesan cheese
2 Tbsp pine nuts
1/8 tsp salt
Freshly ground black pepper, to taste

DIRECTIONS

1. Place haricots verts in a microwave-safe bowl with 1/4 cup water. Cover and cook in the microwave for 4 minutes to steam. Haricots verts should be cooked through but still slightly crisp and bright green in color.

2. While you are steaming the haricots verts, heat olive oil over medium-high heat and sauté shallots for about 3 minutes or until they start to brown.

3. Warm cooked brown rice (according to package directions, if store-bought).

4. In a medium serving bowl, combine brown rice, haricots verts, shallots, Parmesan cheese, pine nuts, salt, and pepper. Mix well and serve warm.

BASIC NUTRITIONAL VALUES	
Calories	**140**
Calories from Fat	50
Total Fat	**6.0 g**
Saturated Fat	0.8 g
Trans Fat	0.0 g
Cholesterol	**0 mg**
Sodium	**95 mg**
Potassium	**190 mg**
Total Carbohydrate	**19 g**
Dietary Fiber	3 g
Sugars	1 g
Protein	**4 g**
Phosphorus	**105 mg**

CHOICES/EXCHANGES

1 Starch, 1 Nonstarchy Vegetable, 1 Fat

Parmesan Mashed Cauliflower

Cauliflower easily replaces potatoes for a lower-carb side dish.

INGREDIENTS

1 medium head cauliflower
6 Tbsp nonfat, plain Greek yogurt
1/4 cup freshly grated Parmesan cheese
1/2 tsp garlic powder
1/4 tsp white pepper
1 Tbsp chopped green onions

Prep Time: 10 minutes
Cook Time: 8 minutes
Serves: 4
Serving Size: 1/2 cup

DIRECTIONS

1. Wash whole cauliflower and cut into florets.
2. Place cauliflower in a microwave-safe dish and microwave for about 8 minutes until cauliflower is soft. Stir halfway through cooking time.
3. Place cauliflower, yogurt, cheese, garlic powder, and white pepper in a food processor or blender and blend until smooth.
4. Top with green onions and serve.

BASIC NUTRITIONAL VALUES

Calories	60
Calories from Fat	20
Total Fat	2.0 g
Saturated Fat	0.9 g
Trans Fat	0.0 g
Cholesterol	2 mg
Sodium	90 mg
Potassium	240 mg
Total Carbohydrate	7 g
Dietary Fiber	3 g
Sugars	4 g
Protein	6 g
Phosphorus	105 mg

CHOICES/EXCHANGES

1 Nonstarchy Vegetable, 1/2 Fat

Peanut Sesame Veggie Stir-Fry

Frozen vegetables cook in minutes and are a time-saving option for a healthful dinner.

INGREDIENTS

1 tsp sesame oil
1 (16-oz) package Asian stir-fry frozen vegetables
9 Tbsp Spicy Peanut Dressing (page 23)

DIRECTIONS

1. Heat sesame oil over medium-high heat in large pan or wok.
2. Add frozen vegetables and cook for about 5 minutes until tender.
3. Add dressing and sauté for an additional 2–3 minutes.

Prep Time: 5 minutes
Cook Time: 10 minutes
Serves: 5
Serving Size: 1/2 cup

BASIC NUTRITIONAL VALUES

Calories	**70**
Calories from Fat	20
Total Fat	**2.0 g**
Saturated Fat	0.3 g
Trans Fat	0.0 g
Cholesterol	**0 mg**
Sodium	**110 mg**
Potassium	**350 mg**
Total Carbohydrate	**10 g**
Dietary Fiber	3 g
Sugars	4 g
Protein	**3 g**
Phosphorus	**90 mg**

CHOICES/EXCHANGES

2 Nonstarchy Vegetable, 1/2 Fat

Pine Nut Olive Couscous

Whole-wheat couscous cooks in minutes, providing an easy whole-grain side dish for weeknight dinners. Experiment with different herbs to create unique flavors.

INGREDIENTS

1 tsp olive oil
1 cup water
1 cup dry whole-wheat couscous
3 Tbsp pine nuts
15 chopped Spanish olives
1/2 cup chopped fresh parsley
2 Tbsp lemon juice
1/2 tsp garlic powder
1/4 tsp freshly ground black pepper

Prep Time: 5 minutes
Cook Time: 5 minutes
Serves: 7
Serving Size: 1/2 cup

DIRECTIONS

1. Add oil to water in a saucepan and bring to a boil. Add couscous, stir, cover, and remove from heat. Keep covered for 5 minutes or until water is absorbed. Remove lid and fluff with a fork.
2. Add remaining ingredients to couscous and serve warm.

BASIC NUTRITIONAL VALUES

Calories	130
Calories from Fat	35
Total Fat	**4.0 g**
Saturated Fat	0.4 g
Trans Fat	0.0 g
Cholesterol	**0 mg**
Sodium	**75 mg**
Potassium	**95 mg**
Total Carbohydrate	**20 g**
Dietary Fiber	3 g
Sugars	1 g
Protein	**4 g**
Phosphorus	**65 mg**

CHOICES/EXCHANGES

1 1/2 Starch, 1/2 Fat

Quick Pan-Cooked Garlic Asparagus

Here's a delicious side that comes together in 10 minutes with minimal prep and chopping! It's great for nights when you're struggling to get a veggie side dish on the table!

INGREDIENTS

1 tsp olive oil
8 oz asparagus, cleaned and trimmed
Freshly ground black pepper, to taste
1 clove garlic, minced
3 Tbsp Pesto Vinaigrette (page 21)
2 tsp shaved Parmesan cheese

Prep Time: 5 minutes
Cook Time: 5 minutes
Serves: 2
Serving Size: 3/4 cup

DIRECTIONS

1. In a large sauté pan, heat oil over medium heat.
2. Add asparagus and pepper and sauté for 4 1/2 minutes, stirring occasionally.
3. Add garlic and sauté for an additional 30 seconds.
4. Remove pan from heat, add vinaigrette and toss.
5. Top each 3/4-cup serving of asparagus with 1 tsp Parmesan cheese and serve warm.

BASIC NUTRITIONAL VALUES

Calories	**100**
Calories from Fat	70
Total Fat	**8.0 g**
Saturated Fat	1.3 g
Trans Fat	0.0 g
Cholesterol	**0 mg**
Sodium	**80 mg**
Potassium	**230 mg**
Total Carbohydrate	**5 g**
Dietary Fiber	2 g
Sugars	1 g
Protein	**3 g**
Phosphorus	**60 mg**

CHOICES/EXCHANGES

1 Nonstarchy Vegetable, 1 1/2 Fat

Quick Veggie and Quinoa Sauté

This nutritious side pairs easily with a fish or chicken entrée—and the colorful veggies combined with the spicy and lemony flavors will make your meal pop!

INGREDIENTS

2 tsp olive oil
1/2 red onion, diced
1 red pepper, diced
1 small zucchini, sliced and cut into half-moons
1 small yellow squash, sliced and cut into half-moons
1 tsp dried basil
Red pepper flakes, to taste
1/8 tsp salt
1 Tbsp pine nuts
1/2 cup cooked quinoa
Juice of 1/2 lemon

Prep Time: 10 minutes
Cook Time: 9 minutes
Serves: 5
Serving Size: 3/4 cup

DIRECTIONS

1. Heat olive oil in a skillet over medium-high heat. Add onion and red pepper and sauté for 2 minutes. Add zucchini, yellow squash, basil, red pepper flakes, and salt and cook, stirring occasionally, for an additional 5–7 minutes or until vegetables are cooked through.
2. Remove pan from heat. Stir in pine nuts and quinoa and drizzle with lemon juice. Serve immediately.

BASIC NUTRITIONAL VALUES

Calories	**90**
Calories from Fat	30
Total Fat	**3.5 g**
Saturated Fat	0.4 g
Trans Fat	0.0 g
Cholesterol	**0 mg**
Sodium	**65 mg**
Potassium	**330 mg**
Total Carbohydrate	**12 g**
Dietary Fiber	3 g
Sugars	5 g
Protein	**2 g**
Phosphorus	**80 mg**

CHOICES/EXCHANGES

2 Nonstarchy Vegetable, 1 Fat

Red Pepper Quinoa

Enjoy this grain and bean salad that is perfect with simple protein entrées at dinnertime and even better for lunch the next day.

INGREDIENTS

1/2 cup dry tricolor quinoa
1 cup water
1/4 cup chopped onion
2 cloves garlic, crushed
1 red pepper, chopped (1 1/2 cups)
2 tsp olive oil
2 cups fresh kale
1/3 cup drained and rinsed white beans (such as cannellini beans)
1/3 cup walnuts
1 Tbsp white cooking wine (or lemon juice)
1 Tbsp balsamic vinegar

Prep Time: 10 minutes
Cook Time: 20 minutes
Serves: 5
Serving Size: 2/3 cup

DIRECTIONS

1. Cook quinoa in water according to package instructions, omitting any added salt.
2. While quinoa is cooking, sauté onion, garlic, and red pepper over medium-high heat in olive oil for about 10 minutes.
3. Add kale and beans to pepper mixture and continue to sauté until kale is wilted, about 5 more minutes.
4. Stir pepper mixture, walnuts, wine (or lemon juice), and balsamic vinegar into the quinoa. Serve warm or cold.

BASIC NUTRITIONAL VALUES

Calories	180
Calories from Fat	70
Total Fat	**8.0 g**
Saturated Fat	0.9 g
Trans Fat	0.0 g
Cholesterol	**0 mg**
Sodium	**20 mg**
Potassium	**360 mg**
Total Carbohydrate	**21 g**
Dietary Fiber	4 g
Sugars	4 g
Protein	**6 g**
Phosphorus	**150 mg**

CHOICES/EXCHANGES

1 Starch, 1 Nonstarchy Vegetable, 1 1/2 Fat

Roasted Brussels Sprouts and Butternut Squash

Roasting veggies brings out their sweetness as they develop a caramelized coating. Try roasting any of your favorite vegetables and experiment with different herbs for variety. To save time when cooking with butternut squash, buy prepackaged squash and cut down larger chunks.

INGREDIENTS

12 oz fresh Brussels sprouts
20 oz butternut squash, cubed (about 3 1/2 cups)
1 Tbsp olive oil
2 tsp dried thyme

DIRECTIONS

1. Preheat oven to 450°F.
2. Slice Brussels sprouts in half. Cut larger pieces of squash into 1-inch cubes.
3. Place sprouts and squash in a large bowl and drizzle with olive oil. Stir in thyme.
4. Place sprouts and squash in a shallow baking pan in 1 layer and bake for 25 minutes.

Prep Time: 10 minutes
Cook Time: 25 minutes
Serves: 7
Serving Size: 1/2 cup

BASIC NUTRITIONAL VALUES

Calories	**60**
Calories from Fat	20
Total Fat	**2.0 g**
Saturated Fat	0.3 g
Trans Fat	0.0 g
Cholesterol	**0 mg**
Sodium	**15 mg**
Potassium	**370 mg**
Total Carbohydrate	**11 g**
Dietary Fiber	4 g
Sugars	2 g
Protein	**2 g**
Phosphorus	**50 mg**

CHOICES/EXCHANGES

1/2 Starch, 1 Nonstarchy Vegetable

Roasted Cauliflower and Red Onion

This simple side makes for perfectly cooked veggies that pair well with roasted or grilled chicken.

INGREDIENTS

Nonstick cooking spray
1 head cauliflower, cut into small florets (about 5 cups florets)
1 medium red onion, sliced into large slices
3 Tbsp olive oil
1/2 tsp freshly ground black pepper
1/4 tsp sea salt

Prep Time: 10 minutes
Cook Time: 40 minutes
Serves: 7
Serving Size: 1/2 cup

DIRECTIONS

1. Preheat oven to 425°F. Line a large baking pan with foil and spray lightly with cooking spray.
2. In a large bowl, toss together cauliflower, onion, and olive oil. Spread vegetable mixture in pan in a single layer.
3. Sprinkle vegetables with pepper and salt and place in the oven. Cook for 40 minutes. Stir veggies 1–2 times during the cooking process.
4. Remove pan from the oven and pull up sides of foil and pinch together to make a packet. Allow veggies to sit for 5 minutes, then serve.

BASIC NUTRITIONAL VALUES

Calories	80
Calories from Fat	50
Total Fat	6.0 g
Saturated Fat	0.9 g
Trans Fat	0.0 g
Cholesterol	0 mg
Sodium	95 mg
Potassium	210 mg
Total Carbohydrate	5 g
Dietary Fiber	2 g
Sugars	2 g
Protein	1 g
Phosphorus	35 mg

CHOICES/EXCHANGES

1 Nonstarchy Vegetable, 1 Fat

Roasted Squash, Broccoli, and Cranberry Medley

This side is a great combination of starchy and nonstarchy vegetables with a touch of sweetness from the dried fruit.

Prep Time: 10 minutes
Cook Time: 25 minutes
Serves: 4
Serving Size: 3/4 cup

INGREDIENTS

Nonstick cooking spray
2 cups cubed butternut squash (about 3/4-inch cubes)
1 large head broccoli, cut into florets (about 4 cups florets)
1 1/2 tsp olive oil
Freshly ground black pepper, to taste
1/4 cup dried cranberries
1/4 tsp salt

DIRECTIONS

1. Preheat oven to 425°F. Line a large baking pan with aluminum foil and spray lightly with cooking spray.

2. Spread butternut squash and broccoli in baking pan in a single layer and drizzle with olive oil. Toss lightly to coat, then season with pepper. Roast in the oven for 25 minutes, stirring once in the middle of cooking.

3. Once vegetables are cooked through and lightly browned, remove the pan from the oven and place vegetables in a serving bowl. Toss in dried cranberries and sprinkle with salt. Serve warm.

BASIC NUTRITIONAL VALUES

Calories	80
Calories from Fat	20
Total Fat	**2.0 g**
Saturated Fat	0.3 g
Trans Fat	0.0 g
Cholesterol	**0 mg**
Sodium	**170 mg**
Potassium	**400 mg**
Total Carbohydrate	**16 g**
Dietary Fiber	4 g
Sugars	8 g
Protein	**3 g**
Phosphorus	**65 mg**

CHOICES/EXCHANGES

1/2 Carbohydrate, 1 Nonstarchy Vegetable, 1/2 Fat

Roasted Sweet Potatoes with Gorgonzola

Looking for a way to spice up your sweet potatoes? Look no further! This recipe makes a tasty side and is also a great option if you're entertaining—especially around the holidays!

INGREDIENTS

Nonstick cooking spray
2 large (10-oz) sweet potatoes, cut into 3/4-inch cubes
1 Tbsp olive oil
1/2 tsp smoked paprika
1 tsp garlic powder
1/2 tsp freshly ground black pepper
1/4 cup gorgonzola cheese

Prep Time: 10 minutes
Cook Time: 30 minutes
Serves: 8
Serving Size: 1/2 cup

DIRECTIONS

1. Preheat oven to 425°F. Line a large baking sheet with aluminum foil and spray lightly with cooking spray.

2. Spread sweet potatoes in one layer on baking sheet and drizzle with olive oil. Toss potatoes with your hands to coat evenly.

3. In a small bowl or ramekin, combine paprika, garlic powder, and pepper. Sprinkle spice mixture over potatoes and roast in the oven for 30 minutes, stirring once at 15 minutes to ensure even cooking.

4. Remove from oven and transfer potatoes to a serving dish. Sprinkle gorgonzola cheese over potatoes and serve immediately.

BASIC NUTRITIONAL VALUES

Calories	**80**
Calories from Fat	25
Total Fat	**3.0 g**
Saturated Fat	1.0 g
Trans Fat	0.0 g
Cholesterol	**3 mg**
Sodium	**80 mg**
Potassium	**290 mg**
Total Carbohydrate	**12 g**
Dietary Fiber	2 g
Sugars	4 g
Protein	**2 g**
Phosphorus	**50 mg**

CHOICES/EXCHANGES

1 Starch, 1/2 Fat

Sautéed Shredded Kale with Golden Raisins

Shredded kale cooks very quickly and pairs perfectly with the savory cooked onions, garlic, and golden raisins in this recipe.

Prep Time: 10 minutes
Cook Time: 6 minutes
Serves: 3
Serving Size: 1 cup

INGREDIENTS

2 tsp olive oil
1 cup finely diced white onion
2 cloves garlic, minced
5 cups shredded kale
1/2 tsp freshly ground black pepper
1/4 tsp sea salt
3 Tbsp golden raisins

DIRECTIONS

1. In a large skillet, heat olive oil over medium-high heat. Add onion and cook for about 3 minutes, until onion begins to turn translucent.
2. Add garlic and cook for another minute. Then add kale and cook for about 2 more minutes or until it turns bright green and begins to wilt.
3. Remove pan from heat and add pepper, sea salt, and raisins. Toss together to fully mix flavors.

BASIC NUTRITIONAL VALUES

Calories	110
Calories from Fat	30
Total Fat	3.5 g
Saturated Fat	0.5 g
Trans Fat	0.0 g
Cholesterol	0 mg
Sodium	200 mg
Potassium	430 mg
Total Carbohydrate	19 g
Dietary Fiber	3 g
Sugars	9 g
Protein	3 g
Phosphorus	80 mg

CHOICES/EXCHANGES

1/2 Fruit, 2 Nonstarchy Vegetable, 1/2 Fat

Simple Sautéed Spinach with Strawberries

You can also try this simple recipe with fresh spinach (instead of frozen) and use any leftover spinach in omelets, soups, or a salad.

Prep Time: 10 minutes
Cook Time: 10 minutes
Serves: 4
Serving Size: 3/4 cup

INGREDIENTS

1 (12-oz) package frozen, chopped spinach
1 Tbsp olive oil
1 cup sliced strawberries
1 Tbsp balsamic vinegar

DIRECTIONS

1. Cook frozen spinach in the microwave according to package instructions. Drain well in a colander.
2. Heat olive oil in a skillet over medium heat.
3. Add spinach to skillet and sauté for about 8 minutes.
4. Add sliced strawberries to skillet and heat for 2 minutes.
5. Remove skillet from heat and drizzle spinach mixture with vinegar.

BASIC NUTRITIONAL VALUES

Calories	70
Calories from Fat	35
Total Fat	4.0 g
Saturated Fat	0.6 g
Trans Fat	0.0 g
Cholesterol	0 mg
Sodium	65 mg
Potassium	270 mg
Total Carbohydrate	7 g
Dietary Fiber	3 g
Sugars	3 g
Protein	3 g
Phosphorus	45 mg

CHOICES/EXCHANGES

1 Nonstarchy Vegetable, 1 Fat

Slaw with Mango and Cilantro Lime Dressing

This tasty salad pairs well with any Mexican-style dish, grilled fish, or chicken!

INGREDIENTS

Cilantro Lime Dressing
1/4 cup light mayonnaise
1/4 cup nonfat, plain Greek yogurt
1/4 cup chopped cilantro
1 tsp lime zest
Juice of 2 limes
1 Tbsp olive oil
1/4 tsp freshly ground black pepper

Salad
1 (14-oz) bag cabbage slaw
1 1/4 cups diced mango
1 cup diced red pepper
1/4 cup chopped cilantro

DIRECTIONS

1. In a small mixing bowl, whisk together all Cilantro Lime Dressing ingredients.
2. In a larger salad bowl, combine all salad ingredients. Top salad with dressing and toss to coat.

Prep Time: 15 minutes
Cook Time: N/A
Serves: 7
Serving Size: 1 cup

BASIC NUTRITIONAL VALUES

Calories	**90**
Calories from Fat	35
Total Fat	**4.0 g**
Saturated Fat	0.5 g
Trans Fat	0.0 g
Cholesterol	**0 mg**
Sodium	**85 mg**
Potassium	**270 mg**
Total Carbohydrate	**12 g**
Dietary Fiber	3 g
Sugars	7 g
Protein	**1 g**
Phosphorus	**35 mg**

CHOICES/EXCHANGES

1/2 Fruit, 1 Nonstarchy Vegetable, 1 Fat

Sweet Marjoram Carrots

Adding fresh herbs like marjoram to simple sides like steamed veggies, rice, or quinoa enhances the flavor and makes the ordinary special.

INGREDIENTS

1 tsp olive oil
2 cloves garlic, chopped
1/4 cup sliced green onions
12 oz carrots (about 56 baby carrots)
2 tsp maple syrup
2 Tbsp fresh marjoram leaves, chopped

Prep Time: 5 minutes
Cook Time: 30 minutes
Serves: 4
Serving Size: 1/2 cup carrots (about 14)

DIRECTIONS

1. Heat oil over medium-high heat in a skillet and sauté garlic and green onions for 4 minutes.
2. Add carrots and stir to evenly coat them.
3. Cover skillet with a lid and steam carrots for about 12 minutes, or until carrots begin to soften.
4. Remove lid and drizzle maple syrup over carrots. Continue to cook for another 10 minutes until carrots begin to brown.
5. Stir in fresh marjoram and heat for 1 minute.

BASIC NUTRITIONAL VALUES

Calories	**60**
Calories from Fat	15
Total Fat	**1.5 g**
Saturated Fat	0.2 g
Trans Fat	0.0 g
Cholesterol	**0 mg**
Sodium	**60 mg**
Potassium	**310 mg**
Total Carbohydrate	**12 g**
Dietary Fiber	3 g
Sugars	6 g
Protein	**1 g**
Phosphorus	**35 mg**

CHOICES/EXCHANGES

2 Nonstarchy Vegetable

Toasted Almond Rice

Lightly toasting nuts brings out their flavor, adding to the richness of this simple side dish.

INGREDIENTS

1 cup dry brown rice
1/4 cup unsalted, sliced toasted almonds
1 tsp grated fresh ginger
2 tsp dried parsley
1/2 tsp freshly ground black pepper

Prep Time: 10 minutes
Cook Time: 30 minutes
Serves: 4
Serving Size: 1/2 cup

DIRECTIONS

1. Cook rice according to package instructions, omitting any added salt.
2. Once rice is cooked, add all other ingredients to the rice and mix well.

BASIC NUTRITIONAL VALUES

Calories	**150**
Calories from Fat	40
Total Fat	**4.5 g**
Saturated Fat	0.4 g
Trans Fat	0.0 g
Cholesterol	**0 mg**
Sodium	**0 mg**
Potassium	**160 mg**
Total Carbohydrate	**23 g**
Dietary Fiber	2 g
Sugars	1 g
Protein	**5 g**
Phosphorus	**140 mg**

CHOICES/EXCHANGES

1 1/2 Starch, 1 Fat

Tropical Quinoa

This is a great side for those who like a little sweet in an otherwise savory dish. It can be served warm or cold.

INGREDIENTS

1/2 cup dry tricolor quinoa
1 Tbsp olive oil
6 cups chopped fresh kale
1/2 (20-oz) can pineapple chunks (about 24 chunks) packed in pineapple juice, drained (juice and remaining pineapple reserved for another recipe)*
2 Tbsp unsweetened, grated coconut
1/4 cup unsalted, slivered almonds
2 green onions, chopped (about 2 Tbsp)
1 Tbsp finely chopped fresh ginger
3 Tbsp freshly squeezed clementine (or orange) juice

Prep Time: 15 minutes
Cook Time: 20 minutes
Serves: 4
Serving Size: 3/4 cup

DIRECTIONS

1. Preheat oven to 350°F.
2. Cook quinoa according to package instructions, omitting any added salt.
3. Heat oil in a nonstick pan over medium-high heat. Sauté kale and pineapple chunks for about 4 minutes.
4. Place coconut and almonds on a baking sheet and toast in the oven for about 6 minutes. Stir every 2 minutes to prevent burning.
5. Combine quinoa and kale mixture with coconut and almonds and the rest of the ingredients. Stir well and serve warm or cold, according to your preference.

*The pineapple juice can be reserved and used in the Pineapple Chile Chicken recipe (page 96), and the remaining half of the pineapple chunks can be used in the Slow-Cooker Almond Rice Pudding recipe (page 85).

BASIC NUTRITIONAL VALUES

Calories	**230**
Calories from Fat	100
Total Fat	**11.0 g**
Saturated Fat	2.4 g
Trans Fat	0.0 g
Cholesterol	**0 mg**
Sodium	**20 mg**
Potassium	**520 mg**
Total Carbohydrate	**30 g**
Dietary Fiber	5 g
Sugars	11 g
Protein	**7 g**
Phosphorus	**185 mg**

CHOICES/EXCHANGES

1 Starch, 1/2 Fruit, 1 Nonstarchy Vegetable, 2 Fat

Pecan Sweet Potato Cups

This dish is a light and fluffy alternative to high-calorie sweet potato casseroles. These potatoes are beautiful to serve for a holiday meal or any time.

INGREDIENTS

1 1/2 lb sweet potatoes
1/2 cup orange juice (no pulp)
1 egg
3/4 tsp baking powder
6 foil muffin cups (or a double layer of paper cups)
1/4 cup chopped pecans

Prep Time: 25 minutes
Cook Time: 30 minutes
Serves: 6
Serving Size: 1 muffin cup

DIRECTIONS

1. Preheat oven to 350°F.
2. Scrub sweet potatoes, poke each sweet potato with fork, and microwave for 8 minutes.
3. Remove skins from microwaved potatoes (skins will remove easily). Discard skins and in a large bowl, beat potatoes with a mixer for at least 5 minutes.
4. Add orange juice and egg. Mix on high for 5 more minutes with a mixer.
5. Add baking powder and mix on high another 5 minutes until mixture is fluffy.
6. Spoon about 1/2 cup mixture into each lined muffin cup. Bake for 15 minutes.
7. Remove from oven and sprinkle pecans on each muffin cup. Return to oven until pecans are toasted, about 5 minutes. Serve immediately.

BASIC NUTRITIONAL VALUES

Calories	**130**
Calories from Fat	40
Total Fat	**4.5 g**
Saturated Fat	0.6 g
Trans Fat	0.0 g
Cholesterol	**30 mg**
Sodium	**85 mg**
Potassium	**460 mg**
Total Carbohydrate	**20 g**
Dietary Fiber	3 g
Sugars	7 g
Protein	**3 g**
Phosphorus	**135 mg**

CHOICES/EXCHANGES

1 1/2 Starch, 1/2 Fat

Black Bean and Caramelized Onion Quinoa

Caramelizing onions brings out the sweetness in the onion that is a key to this dish. It requires patience, but the long cook time is worth the wait!

Prep Time: 10 minutes
Cook Time: 50 minutes
Serves: 7
Serving Size: 3/4 cup

INGREDIENTS

1/2 cup dry tricolor quinoa
1 cup water
2 cups chopped red onion
1 Tbsp olive oil
1 (15.5-oz) can black beans, drained and rinsed
8 oz grape tomatoes, sliced in half
1/2 cup fresh parsley
1/2 tsp red pepper flakes
1/2 cup crumbled feta cheese

DIRECTIONS

1. Cook quinoa in water according to package directions.
2. In a skillet, sauté onion in olive oil for about 40 minutes. Stir often to prevent burning, but allow onions to get brown.
3. Add beans, cooked quinoa, tomatoes, parsley, and red pepper flakes to the skillet. Gently stir in feta.
4. Can serve warm or cold.

BASIC NUTRITIONAL VALUES

Calories	**160**
Calories from Fat	40
Total Fat	**4.5 g**
Saturated Fat	1.6 g
Trans Fat	0.1 g
Cholesterol	**5 mg**
Sodium	**140 mg**
Potassium	**370 mg**
Total Carbohydrate	**23 g**
Dietary Fiber	5 g
Sugars	5 g
Protein	**7 g**
Phosphorus	**155 mg**

CHOICES/EXCHANGES

1 Starch, 1 Nonstarchy
Vegetable, 1 Fat

Fried Green Tomatoes

This is a lighter version of a southern favorite with all the flavor of the traditional dish.

INGREDIENTS

2 large (7-oz) green tomatoes
1/4 cup cornmeal
1/2 tsp garlic powder
1/4 tsp freshly ground black pepper
1 Tbsp parsley
1/4 tsp salt
1 egg
1 Tbsp nonfat milk
2 Tbsp olive oil

Prep Time: 10 minutes
Cook Time: 20 minutes
Serves: 5
Serving Size: 2 slices

DIRECTIONS

1. Slice tomatoes into 5 slices each.
2. Mix cornmeal, garlic powder, pepper, parsley, and salt together in a small bowl.
3. In a separate bowl, whisk egg and milk together.
4. Dredge tomato slices through egg mixture and then coat with cornmeal mixture.
5. Heat olive oil in a skillet over medium heat. Add tomato slices and cook each side until tomato is soft on inside and coating is golden brown.

BASIC NUTRITIONAL VALUES

Calories	**110**
Calories from Fat	60
Total Fat	**7.0 g**
Saturated Fat	1.1 g
Trans Fat	0.0 g
Cholesterol	**35 mg**
Sodium	**140 mg**
Potassium	**190 mg**
Total Carbohydrate	**10 g**
Dietary Fiber	1 g
Sugars	3 g
Protein	**3 g**
Phosphorus	**50 mg**

CHOICES/EXCHANGES

1/2 Starch, 1 Nonstarchy Vegetable, 1 Fat

Garlic-Thyme Roasted Mushrooms and Carrots

This simple roasted vegetable dish packs tons of flavor and requires minimal prep. You can jazz up the look of this veggie side by using tricolor carrots, usually available in grocery stores during the colder months.

INGREDIENTS

Nonstick cooking spray
8 oz mushrooms, sliced
16 oz baby carrots, cut in half lengthwise
4 cloves garlic, peeled and halved
1 1/2 Tbsp olive oil
1 tsp fresh thyme
Freshly ground black pepper, to taste

Prep Time: 5 minutes
Cook Time: 30 minutes
Serves: 4
Serving Size: 3/4 cup

DIRECTIONS

1. Preheat oven to 450°F, then coat a foil-lined baking sheet with cooking spray and set aside.
2. In a large mixing bowl, combine mushrooms, carrots, and garlic. Drizzle with olive oil and toss to coat veggies. Add thyme and pepper and toss to coat.
3. Spread vegetables in a single layer on the baking sheet and bake for 15 minutes.

4. Remove from oven and stir. Then place back in oven and cook for 10–15 more minutes or until vegetables have begun to brown and caramelize.

Tip: When the veggies are done cooking, remove them from the oven, pull the sides of the foil together, and crimp the foil to make a pouch so the flavors can continue to infuse. Let the foil pouch sit for about 10 minutes and then enjoy!

BASIC NUTRITIONAL VALUES

Calories	110
Calories from Fat	50
Total Fat	**6.0 g**
Saturated Fat	0.8 g
Trans Fat	0.0 g
Cholesterol	**0 mg**
Sodium	**80 mg**
Potassium	**560 mg**
Total Carbohydrate	**14 g**
Dietary Fiber	4 g
Sugars	7 g
Protein	**3 g**
Phosphorus	**95 mg**

CHOICES/EXCHANGES

3 Nonstarchy Vegetable, 1 Fat

Green Beans with Walnuts

Nuts can be used in many basic vegetable dishes to add flavor, texture, and a dose of healthy fats.

INGREDIENTS

8 oz fresh green beans (about 3 cups)
1 tsp olive oil
2 cloves garlic, minced
1/4 cup chopped walnuts
1 Tbsp lemon juice

Prep Time: 5 minutes
Cook Time: 12 minutes
Serves: 4
Serving Size: 1/2 cup

DIRECTIONS

1. Place green beans in a microwave-safe dish. Microwave for 2 minutes.
2. In a skillet, heat olive oil over medium heat and sauté garlic for 2 minutes.
3. Add green beans and sauté for 6 minutes. Add walnuts and sauté for another 2 minutes.
4. Sprinkle with lemon juice and serve.

BASIC NUTRITIONAL VALUES

Calories	**80**
Calories from Fat	50
Total Fat	**6.0 g**
Saturated Fat	0.6 g
Trans Fat	0.0 g
Cholesterol	**0 mg**
Sodium	**0 mg**
Potassium	**115 mg**
Total Carbohydrate	**6 g**
Dietary Fiber	2 g
Sugars	1 g
Protein	**2 g**
Phosphorus	**45 mg**

CHOICES/EXCHANGES

1 Nonstarchy Vegetable, 1 Fat

SUPERFOOD-PACKED
MEAL PLANS

You may be thinking to yourself, "Recipes are great, but what do I serve with them?" Look no further than the 40 days of meal plans in this chapter, which show you how to incorporate our recipes into your day. Each meal plan includes at least 2 of our superfood recipes, plus additional superfoods and quick ideas to provide balanced meals and snacks.

To create these meal plans, we followed very general diabetes nutrition guidelines from the American Diabetes Association (see Our Meal Planning Guidelines below). Rather than creating meals and snacks that fall within specific ranges of calories and carbohydrates, these meal plans can be customized to meet your individual nutrition needs. You may need more or less of certain nutrients depending on your health status and other conditions and factors. For example, if you have high blood pressure, you may need to restrict sodium more than our meal plan suggests. Every person has different needs when it comes to nutrition.

You'll see that these meal plans do not include serving sizes for the foods listed, and we do not provide nutrition information for each plan. Instead, you can enjoy the foods in these meal plans in the serving sizes that fit with *your personal meal plan*. A guide for the serving amount is included with the recipe, and you can always use the Diabetes Plate Method (see pages xiv–xv) as a guide. You may need to eat more or less of the foods listed depending on your calorie and carbohydrate needs. The goal of these meal plans is to help you incorporate flavorful, nutritious diabetes superfoods into your meals and snacks in a way that works best for you.

Our Meal Planning Guidelines:

- Each meal plan includes breakfast, lunch, dinner, and one snack.
- Meal plans are designed so leftovers can be used the next day for other meals.
- In order to minimize your trips to the grocery store, the meal plans purposefully use ingredients more than once in any given week.
- Fruits or vegetables are included at every meal and most snacks.

WHAT IS A MEAL PLAN?

A meal plan is a guide that tells you how much and what kinds of food to choose at meals and snack times. Some people may refer to a meal plan as an eating plan, food plan, menu, or diet. All of these terms essentially mean the same thing. Your plan should be created with the help of your diabetes care team and should fit your schedule, culture, and food preferences. The right plan should help you manage your blood glucose and meet your health goals.

- The calories and carbohydrates in each plan will depend on how much you eat of the foods listed.
  - There is no one amount of calories or carbohydrate that is best for everyone with diabetes. Work with your healthcare provider, dietitian, or certified diabetes educator to determine your personal calorie and carbohydrate needs.
- Plans limit trans fat as much as possible, limit saturated fat, and focus on healthy fat sources.
  - People with diabetes have a higher-than-average risk of having a heart attack or stroke. Due to this increased risk for heart disease, the amount of saturated and trans fats in our meal plans is limited. Trans fat and saturated fats are sometimes referred to as "unhealthy" fats.
  - A good goal for many people with diabetes is to eat less than 10 percent of calories from saturated fat and avoid trans fats whenever possible.
  - Healthy fats include monounsaturated and polyunsaturated fats and may promote heart health. Meal plans include these over "unhealthy" fats as much as possible.
- Plans were designed to provide a significant amount of dietary fiber to help you reach the recommended daily amount.
  - You get fiber from plant-based foods like whole grains, fruit, vegetables, nuts, seeds, and beans.
  - It is recommended that women consume at least 25 grams of dietary fiber per day and men consume at least 38 grams per day. Many Americans only get about half the recommended amount.
- Plans limit sodium to help you stay within the daily amount recommended by the American Diabetes Association.
  - The American Diabetes Association recommends 2,300 mg of sodium or less per day.
  - If you have diabetes and hypertension, you should work with your healthcare team to see if further reduction of sodium intake is necessary.

> Remember, although the meal plans in this book were designed with the general nutrition guidelines of the American Diabetes Association in mind, we encourage you to work with your healthcare provider, a registered dietitian, or a certified diabetes educator to build a plan that is individualized for you and will help you meet your diabetes management goals.

Meal Plan

WEEK 1

MEAL	DAY 1	DAY 2	DAY 3	DAY 4	DAY 5
Breakfast	Mini Red Pepper and Mushroom Frittatas Small orange 100% whole-wheat toast with: ■ Trans fat–free margarine Coffee or tea	Mini Red Pepper and Mushroom Frittatas Nonfat, plain Greek yogurt with: ■ Banana ■ Drizzle of honey Coffee or tea	Nonfat, vanilla Greek yogurt Strawberries Chopped walnuts Coffee or tea	Nonfat, plain Greek yogurt with: ■ 1/2 banana ■ Fresh mango slices Dry-roasted almonds (unsalted) Coffee or tea	100% whole-wheat toast with: ■ Avocado ■ Freshly ground black pepper, to taste Small orange Coffee or tea
Lunch	Salad made with: ■ Spinach ■ White beans ■ Diced cucumber ■ Quinoa ■ Homemade Balsamic Dressing ■ Chopped walnuts Red grapes Sparkling water	Simple Salmon Salad Peach 100% whole-wheat crackers Water	Chicken Salad Sliders Small orange Cucumber slices Lemony Pesto Hummus Sparkling water	Chicken Salad Sliders Peach Sliced red pepper Sparkling water	Hard-boiled egg Small apple 100% whole-wheat crackers Baby carrots Lemony Pesto Hummus Water
Dinner	Simple Roasted Salmon Farro, Tomato, and Basil Salad Skim milk	Rotisserie chicken (no salt added) Farro, Tomato, and Basil Salad served over: ■ Spinach Skim milk	Shrimp Fried Cauliflower Rice Steamed sugar snap peas with: ■ Trans fat–free margarine ■ Freshly ground black pepper, to taste Diced mango Water	Crispy Polenta with Veggies and White Beans Strawberries Skim milk	Turkey Tacos Slaw with Mango and Cilantro Lime Dressing Water
Snack	Small apple Peanut or almond butter	Lemony Pesto Hummus Baby carrots	Nonfat, plain Greek yogurt Blueberries Baby carrots	Sugar snap peas Light popcorn	Small apple Dry-roasted almonds (unsalted)

Meal Plan

MEAL	DAY 1	DAY 2	DAY 3	DAY 4	DAY 5
Breakfast	Nonfat, plain Greek yogurt Blueberries Raspberries Coffee or tea	Savory Quinoa Breakfast Bowls Coffee or tea	Pumpkin Overnight Oats Small banana Hard-boiled egg Coffee or tea	Pumpkin Overnight Oats Blueberries Hard-boiled egg Coffee or tea	Open-Faced Egg Sandwiches Orange Coffee or tea
Lunch	Turkey wrap made with: ■ Low-carb wheat tortilla ■ Roma tomato, sliced ■ Greens ■ Low-sodium deli turkey breast ■ Light mayo Clementine Sparkling water	Mediterranean Chicken Pita Green grapes Sugar snap peas Water	Mediterranean Chicken Pita Blueberries Sugar snap peas Water	Cheese and Bean Quesadilla made with: ■ Whole-wheat tortilla ■ Reduced-fat sharp cheddar cheese ■ Reduced-sodium black beans, drained and rinsed ■ Diced tomatoes Nonfat, plain Greek yogurt Green grapes Sparkling water	Butternut Squash and Kale Soup Salad made with: ■ Spinach ■ Avocado ■ White beans ■ Chopped walnuts Water
Dinner	Greek Yogurt–Marinated Grilled Chicken Garlic-Thyme Roasted Mushrooms and Carrots Green grapes Skim milk	Veggie Baked Ziti Salad made with: ■ Greens ■ Diced tomatoes ■ White beans ■ Olive oil and red wine vinegar dressing Water	Baked tilapia with: ■ Freshly ground black pepper, to taste ■ Lemon juice Brown rice Sautéed Shredded Kale with Golden Raisins Skim milk	Pecan-Crusted Pork Tenderloin with Apples and Onions Butternut Squash and Kale Soup Skim milk	Pan-Seared Scallops with Vegetable Ribbons Brown rice with: ■ Freshly ground black pepper, to taste ■ Salt Skim milk
Snack	Dry-roasted almonds (unsalted) Light popcorn	Pumpkin Hummus Baby carrots Celery sticks	Dried fruit and nut mix	Dried fruit and nut mix	Pumpkin Hummus Baby carrots Celery sticks

Meta Plan

MEAL	WEEK 3				
	DAY 1	DAY 2	DAY 3	DAY 4	DAY 5
Breakfast	Southwest Tofu Scramble Mixed berries Coffee or tea	Southwest Tofu Scramble Clementine Coffee or tea	100% whole-wheat English muffin with: ■ Tahini Sauce ■ Roma tomato, sliced ■ Freshly ground black pepper, to taste Hard-boiled egg Coffee or tea	100% whole-wheat English muffin with: ■ Sliced avocado ■ Freshly ground black pepper, to taste Dried apricots Coffee or tea	Open-Faced Egg Sandwiches 100% orange juice Coffee or tea
Lunch	Hard-boiled egg Apple slices Sugar snap peas with: ■ Tahini Sauce Part-skim mozzarella cheese stick Sparkling water	Edamame Veggie Wrap Nonfat, vanilla Greek yogurt with: ■ Toasted walnuts ■ Kiwi, peeled and sliced Water	Nonfat, plain Greek yogurt with: ■ Mixed berries ■ Chopped walnuts Steamed broccoli with: ■ Trans fat–free margarine ■ Freshly ground black pepper, to taste Sparkling water	Slow-Cooker Beef Tacos Greens with: ■ Diced cucumber ■ Olive oil ■ Balsamic vinager Apple slices Water	Grain Bowl made with (leftovers): ■ Quinoa ■ Garbanzo beans ■ Arugula ■ Thinly sliced red onion ■ Cherry tomatoes, halved ■ Pesto Vinaigrette Nonfat, flavored Greek yogurt Sparkling water
Dinner	Quinoa, Arugula, and Apricot Salad Grilled chicken Steamed green beans Water	Slow-Cooker Beef Tacos Super Green Salad Skim milk	Tilapia with Pesto Vinaigrette and Tomatoes Roasted or grilled summer squash and zucchini Cherries Water	Grain Bowl made with: ■ Quinoa ■ Garbanzo beans ■ Arugula ■ Thinly sliced red onion ■ Cherry tomatoes, halved ■ Pesto Vinaigrette Clementine Water	Spinach, Avocado, and Summer Berry Salad Lemon Garlic Grilled Shrimp Corn on the cob Fruit salad Water or an adult beverage (if desired) *Summer cookout menu
Snack	Baby carrots Peanut butter	Banana Cinnamon "Fro-Yo" Mixed berries	Peanut Butter and Oatmeal Energy Bites Baby carrots	Peanut Butter and Oatmeal Energy Bites Sugar snap peas	Whole-wheat pita Sliced cucumbers Roasted Red Pepper Spread

Meal Plan

WEEK 4

	DAY 1	DAY 2	DAY 3	DAY 4	DAY 5
Breakfast	On-the-Go PB&J Oatmeal Banana Coffee or tea	Scrambled egg Orange 100% whole-wheat toast with: ■ Avocado slices Coffee or tea	100% whole-wheat English muffin with: ■ Peanut butter Orange Nonfat cafe latté	100% whole-wheat English muffin with: ■ Cinnamon Almond Butter Dip Grapefruit Coffee or tea	Grapefruit Nonfat, vanilla Greek yogurt Dry-roasted almonds (unsalted) Coffee or tea
Lunch	Hearty Turkey, Poblano, and Pumpkin Chili with: ■ Nonfat, plain Greek yogurt ■ Diced avocado Small apple Water	Hearty Turkey, Poblano, and Pumpkin Chili with: ■ Shredded reduced-fat sharp cheddar cheese Red grapes Water	Veggie wrap made with: ■ Low-carb tortilla ■ Greens ■ Diced tomato ■ Pumpkin Hummus ■ Shredded reduced-fat sharp cheddar cheese ■ Sliced toasted almonds Red grapes Sparkling water	Tuna salad sandwich made with: ■ 100% whole-wheat bread ■ Tuna salad (made with light mayo) ■ Lettuce Small apple Cucumber slices Water	Chicken Tortilla Soup Part-skim mozzarella cheese stick Red grapes Water
Dinner	Chicken Stroganoff Roasted Brussels sprouts Red grapes Water	Roasted salmon made with: ■ Olive oil Roasted Sweet Potatoes with Gorgonzola Greens with: ■ Diced tomato ■ Sliced toasted almonds ■ Homemade oil and vinegar dressing Water	Chicken Stroganoff Roasted Squash, Broccoli, and Cranberry Medley Skim milk Water	Spinach and Turkey Meatballs with: ■ Zucchini noodles or ribbons ■ Lower-sodium marinara sauce Skim milk	Black Bean Quinoa Cakes over Mixed Greens Diced mango Sparkling water
Snack	Light popcorn Banana	Cinnamon Almond Butter Dip Sliced pear	4-Ingredient Guacamole Raw nonstarchy vegetables (celery, endive, carrots) Light popcorn	Pumpkin Hummus Carrots	Lemon Raspberry Chia Seed Pudding

Meal Plan

WEEK 5

MEAL	DAY 1	DAY 2	DAY 3	DAY 4	DAY 5
Breakfast	100% whole-wheat English muffin with: ■ Peanut butter Clementine Milk Coffee or tea	Oatmeal with: ■ Walnuts ■ Dried cranberries ■ Unsweetened vanilla almond milk Coffee or tea	Pecan Sweet Potato Cups Hard-boiled egg Nonfat, plain Greek yogurt with: ■ Sliced strawberries Coffee or tea	Oatmeal with: ■ Chopped peach ■ Dash of cinnamon ■ Chopped pecans Coffee or tea	Fried Egg with Spinach 100% whole-wheat toast with: ■ Mashed avocado Strawberries Coffee or tea
Lunch	Garbanzo Bean and Arugula Salad Nonfat, plain Greek yogurt with: ■ Finely chopped apple with cinnamon Water	Garbanzo Bean and Arugula Salad Clementine 100% whole-wheat crackers Sparkling water	Spicy Peanut Broccoli Slaw Rotisserie chicken (no salt added) Apple Unsweetened iced tea	Whole-wheat wrap with: ■ Spicy Peanut Broccoli Slaw ■ White beans Grapes Water	Italian Stuffed Green Peppers Whole-wheat pasta with: ■ Simple Garlic Marinara Sauce Orange Sparkling Water
Dinner	Eggplant, Quinoa, and Turkey Meat Loaf (freeze leftovers) **Green Beans with Walnuts** Steamed cauliflower Sparkling water	Pecan Sweet Potato Cups Steamed broccoli Grilled salmon with: ■ Freshly ground black pepper, to taste ■ Olive oil Strawberries Unsweetened iced tea	Mixed Greens with Spicy Pecans, Goat Cheese, and Pear Leftover grilled salmon Whole-wheat roll with: ■ Whipped butter Skim milk Water	Italian Stuffed Green Peppers Whole-wheat spaghetti with: ■ Simple Garlic Marinara Sauce Salad made with: ■ Mixed greens ■ Shredded carrot ■ Cherry tomatoes ■ Balsamic dressing Water	Honey Lime Chicken Brown rice Broccoli and cauliflower frozen vegetables, steamed Skim milk Water
Snack	Almonds (unsalted) Light popcorn	Grapes Light cheddar cheese	Nonfat cottage cheese Small peach, chopped	Baby carrots Peanut butter Light popcorn	Honey Spiced Pecans Small apple

Meal Plan

WEEK 6

	DAY 1	DAY 2	DAY 3	DAY 4	DAY 5
Breakfast	Zucchini Quinoa Fritters with Feta Nonfat, plain Greek yogurt with: ■ Mixed berries Coffee or tea	Cauliflower Hash Browns **Breakfast Pepper Sauté** Skim milk Coffee or tea	Sunflower Granola with: ■ Unsweetened vanilla almond milk Orange Coffee or tea	100% whole-wheat English muffin with: ■ Peanut butter Banana Skim milk Coffee or tea	Breakfast Tacos Strawberries Coffee or tea
Lunch	Turkey sandwich made with: ■ Low-sodium deli turkey breast ■ Whole-wheat sandwich thin ■ Sliced avocado ■ Sliced tomato ■ Spinach Apple Unsweetened iced tea	Zucchini Quinoa Fritters with Feta Mixed greens with: ■ Garbanzo beans ■ Cherry tomatoes ■ Cucumber slices ■ Sesame seeds ■ Balsamic dressing Water	Curried Tuna Salad Small orange Whole-wheat pretzels Unsweetened iced tea	Curried Tuna Salad with: ■ Whole-wheat sandwich thin Orange Sparkling water	Sweet Potato Black Bean Chili with: ■ Nonfat, plain Greek yogurt ■ Sliced avocado Orange Water
Dinner	Sesame Ginger Fried Tofu with Broccoli **Toasted Almond Rice** Water	Grilled tilapia made with: ■ Squeeze of lemon ■ Freshly ground black pepper, to taste **Simple Sautéed Spinach with Strawberries** **Toasted Almond Rice** Steamed carrots Sparkling water	Eggplant, Quinoa, and Turkey Meat Loaf (from freezer—left over from previous week) **Quick Cinnamon Baked Apple** with: ■ Yogurt Topping Unsweetened iced tea	Sweet Potato Black Bean Chili with: ■ Nonfat, plain Greek yogurt ■ Sliced avocado Apple Water	Roasted Brussels Sprouts and Butternut Squash Grilled chicken Spinach with: ■ Chopped tomato ■ Shredded carrots ■ Balsamic dressing Sparkling water
Snack	Pistachios (unsalted) Orange	**Quick Cinnamon Baked Apple** Chopped walnuts	100% whole-wheat crackers Almond butter	Light popcorn Pistachios (unsalted)	Apple Peanut butter

Meal Plan

WEEK 7

	DAY 1	DAY 2	DAY 3	DAY 4	DAY 5
Breakfast	100% whole-wheat toast with: ■ Mashed avocado Nonfat, plain Greek yogurt with: ■ Blueberries ■ Honey Coffee or tea	Oatmeal Pecan Pancakes with: ■ **Blueberry Sauce** Coffee or tea	Red pepper half filled with: ■ Nonfat cottage cheese Blueberries Coffee or tea	Orange Ginger Hot Tea Hard-boiled egg, sliced Whole-wheat tortilla with: ■ Spinach ■ Refried beans ■ Salsa ■ Mashed avocado	Oatmeal with: ■ Almonds (unsalted) ■ Strawberries ■ Unsweetened vanilla almond milk Coffee or tea
Lunch	Hard-boiled egg Celery and carrot sticks 100% whole-wheat crackers with: ■ Peanut butter Orange Unsweetened iced tea	**Black Bean and Caramelized Onion Quinoa** Nonfat, plain Greek yogurt with: ■ **Blueberry Sauce** Pecans Sparkling water	Brown rice bowl made with: ■ Brown rice ■ Avocado ■ Salsa ■ Vegetarian refried beans ■ Chopped spinach (wilt under hot rice) ■ Nonfat, plain Greek yogurt ■ Shredded sharp cheddar cheese Orange Water	Whole-wheat sandwich thin with: ■ Peanut butter Banana Baby carrots Skim milk	**Mushroom Arugula Pizza** Baby carrots Cherry tomatoes Clementine Mixed nuts (unsalted) Water
Dinner	**Spicy Slow-Cooker Chicken** **Pine Nut Olive Couscous** Steamed broccoli Water	**Spicy Slow-Cooker Chicken** Brown rice Spinach salad made with: ■ Spinach ■ Chopped turkey bacon ■ Shredded carrots ■ Balsamic dressing Sparkling water	**Sweet Marjoram Carrots** Grilled Tuna made with: ■ Olive oil ■ Lemon pepper seasoning **Black Bean and Caramelized Onion Quinoa** Water	**Parmesan Mashed Cauliflower** Roasted turkey breast **Sweet Marjoram Carrots** Strawberries Skim milk	**Fig and Walnut Yogurt Tarts** **Bruschetta-Stuffed Mushrooms** Guacamole with: ■ Whole-corn tortilla chips Hummus with: ■ Baby carrots *This is a great finger food menu for parties.
Snack	100% whole-wheat crackers Light spreadable cheese wedge (such as Laughing Cow)	**Slow-Cooker Almond Rice Pudding**	Cashews (unsalted) Small apple	**Slow-Cooker Almond Rice Pudding**	Sweet Potato Fries with: ■ **Rosemary Honey Mustard Dipping Sauce**

Meal Plan

MEAL	DAY 1	DAY 2	DAY 3	DAY 4	DAY 5
Breakfast	Spiced Cranberry Hot Tea 100% whole-wheat English muffin with: ■ Almond butter Hard-boiled egg Nonfat, vanilla Greek yogurt	Pumpkin Flaxseed Pancakes with: ■ Strawberry Maple Topping Coffee or tea	Parmesan Grits Fried egg made with: ■ Olive oil ■ Freshly ground black pepper, to taste Sliced tomato Grapefruit Coffee or tea	Oatmeal with: ■ Chopped walnuts ■ Dried cranberries ■ Unsweetened vanilla almond milk Coffee or tea	Grapefruit 100% whole-wheat toast with: ■ Peanut butter Skim milk Coffee or tea
Lunch	Open-faced salmon sandwich made with: ■ 100% whole-wheat English muffin ■ Canned salmon ■ Mayo ■ Freshly ground black pepper, to taste ■ Sliced tomato ■ Sliced onion ■ Romaine lettuce Clementine Sparkling water	Artichoke and Tomato Salad **Pineapple Chile Chicken** with: ■ Corn tortillas ■ Peach salsa ■ Mashed avocado Unsweetened iced tea	100% whole-wheat crackers with: ■ Light spreadable cheese wedge (such as Laughing Cow) Hummus with: ■ Baby carrots ■ Sugar snap peas Mango Water	Red Pepper Quinoa Orange Part-skim mozzarella cheese stick Sparkling water	Mango Freeze Whole-wheat pita with: ■ Shredded Slow-Cooker Roast Chicken (left over from previous night) ■ Spring mix lettuce ■ Sliced tomatoes ■ Cucumber Dill Dip Water
Dinner	Pineapple Chile Chicken **Tropical Quinoa** Steamed carrots Milk Sparkling water	Peanut Sesame Veggie Stir-Fry Brown rice Grilled tuna made with: ■ Freshly ground black pepper, to taste ■ Olive oil Strawberries Water	Red Pepper Quinoa Spring mix salad greens **Artichoke and Tomato Salad** **Chocolate-Dipped Walnuts and Apricots** Decaf coffee Water	Slow-Cooker Roast Chicken and Root Vegetables Shredded romaine lettuce with: ■ Caesar dressing ■ Fresh shaved Parmesan cheese Water	Slow-Cooker Roast Chicken and Root Vegetables **Fried Green Tomatoes** Unsweetened iced tea
Snack	Carrot sticks Sugar snap peas Part-skim mozzarella cheese stick	**Chocolate-Dipped Walnuts and Apricots**	Light popcorn Brazil nuts **Raspberry Mint–Infused Water**	Cucumber Dill Dip Guacamole with: ■ Baby carrots ■ Cauliflower florets	Pistachios (unsalted) Apple

Index